All rights reserved. No part of this book may be reproduced, stored in a retrieval system, or transmitted in any form or by any means, without the prior written permission of the author, except in the case of brief quotations embedded in critical articles or reviews.

Introduction

Hello to all pregnant ladies and expecting dads. I am proud to present you this book, which will definitely help you choose the most suitable, unique, and beautiful name for your baby.

This book is not just another list of a million+ baby names with one word as a description. In this material, I collected only the most unusual, nontrivial, noble, "exotic" and beautiful names, and tried to describe in detail the history of their origin and their meaning.

Have a great time.

Names for Boys

Aaron is a male given name of Hebrew origin meaning "high mountain; exalted, enlightened".

Abel is a male given name of Hebrew origin meaning "breath". In Arabic however, it is derived from the word *habeel* (meaning "a city in mourning"). Abel was the second son of Adam and Eve in the Bible.

Abraham is a male given name of Hebrew origin meaning "father of a multitude of nations".

Adrian is a male given name of Latin origin meaning "from Hadria". There is a town in Italy called Hadria and it is believed that the name was originally applied as a surname to people from there.

Adam is a male given name of Hebrew origin meaning "son of the red earth".

Aidan (AY-dən), *Aiden* and *Aedan* are the main anglicisations of the Irish male given name *Aodhán* and the Scottish Gaelic given name *Aodhàn*. The main meaning is "little fire" or "fiery one."

Ajax is a given name derived from the Greek *Aias*, perhaps deriving from Greek *aiastes* (mourner) or *aia* (earth, land). The name is borne in Greek mythology by two Greeks renowned for their valor and prowess. *Ajax Telamon* (Ajax the Great) was a strong and brave warrior who led the Greeks in the Trojan War after Achilles withdrew. *Ajax the Lesser*, one of the swiftest runners in the Greek Army, was the leader of the Locrian contingent during the Trojan War and a significant figure in Homer's Iliad.

Alaric is a male given name, the Anglicized version of the Germanic name *Alareiks*, meaning "ruler or king".

Albus is a male given name of Latin origin meaning "white, bright".

Alistair is the Scottish form of *Alexander*. Alexander is the Latinized form of the ancient Greek name *Alexandros* (*alexein* (meaning "to defend") + *andros* (meaning "man, warrior" in the possessive) and so specifically means: "defender of mankind"). Adopted by the lowland Scots by the seventeenth century, the name didn't become popular outside Scotland and Ireland until the twentieth century.

Alonso is the Spanish and Portuguese diminutive version of *Alfonso*, itself deriving from an old Germanic name *Adalfuns* (meaning "ready for battle"). Although the Italian spelling *Alonzo* is more popular in the US, Alonso has its own strong history (Alonso Quijano, for example, is the real name of Miguel de Cervantes' famous character "Don Quixote", written in the early 1600s.)

Alvaro (AL-vah-roh) is a Spanish and Portuguese masculine name borrowed from the Germanic language (rather than Latin). Its origins can be found in the Old Norse *Alfarr* (from the components *alfr* (elf) and *arr* (army)). Some etymologists believe that the English *Oliver* may be derived from the same Germanic root elements. *Álvaro* was the name borne by 14 Kings of Kongo between 1568 and 1896.

Amir (a-MEER) is a male given name of Arabic origin that means "prince" or "ruler." In the United States, the name Amir is used primarily among those of Middle Eastern descent. While the name is common among Arabs and Muslims, it is not generally used by English-speaking nations.

Amit is a male given name of Sanskrit origin meanings "endless".

Anders (AN-ders) is the Scandinavian form of *Andrew*, which are both ultimately derived from the Greek *andros* (man, manly, warrior).

Anderson is a male given name of Scandinavian origin meaning "son of Anders".

Angus (ANG-guss) is the Anglicized form of an Old Gaelic name *Aonghus*, a name traditionally used among the Irish and Scottish Gaels, particularly the Scots. The name means "one force", "one strength", or "one of excellence", depending on the translation. It is also sometimes said to mean "one choice." The feminine form of Angus is *Angusina*.

Apollo is a male given name of unknown meaning meaning "strength". Another theory states that Apollo can be equated with *Appaliunas*, an

Anatolian god whose name possibly means "father lion" or "father light".

Aramis (AIR-a-miss) is a male given name taken from Alexandre Dumas's "The Three Musketeers"; Aramis characterized as a famous swordsman, notable for his ambition and religious aspirations.

Archibald is the Modern English and Scottish form of an Old High German name *Ercanbald* derived from the elements *ercan* (genuine) and *bald* (bold). In medieval Europe, the name's meaning was meant to signify the strength and solidity of one's Christian faith.

The name was later altered with the Greek prefix *archos* (meaning "master"). The Norman French brought the name to England after the Conquest of 1066 where it proved most popular among the Scots (particularly the clans Campbell and Douglas).

Arthur is a male given name that was formed through a combination of *artos* (meaning bear), *viros* (meaning man), and *rigos* (meaning king).

Asher is a male given name of Hebrew origin meaning "fortunate, blessed, happy one". In the Bible, Asher was one of Jacob's twelve sons who gave their names to the tribes of Israel.

Athelstan is a given name of Old English origin that means "noble stone." It was the name of King Athelstan the Glorious of England who reigned from 924 - 940 AD. He was the first king of a united England and obtained the submission of the Welsh and Scots.

Atticus (AT-a-kuss) is an old Roman (Latin) name meaning "man of Attica." Attica is a place name; dating back to Antiquity, it is the region in Greece which surrounds Athens. The name was made most famous by author Harper Lee as the protagonist of her 1960 novel, "To Kill a Mockingbird."

August (AW-gust) is both a given name and surname developed from the Latin *Augustus* (derived from the Latin word *augere* (to increase)). Augustus had the meaning "esteemed, great, or venerable" and was a title given to Roman emperors. August is also the eighth month of the calendar year.

Augusto is a male given name of Latin origin meaning "deserving respect".

Aurelio is a male given name of Latin origin meaning "gilded" or "golden".

Austin is a male given name of Latin origin meaning "exalted". It is a short form of *Augustine* (an English variant of *Augustus*).

Avery is a male given name of Old English origin meaning "ruler of elves" (derived from the Old English words *aelf* (meaning "elf") and *ric* (meaning "king or power").

Baker is a male given name that comes from the Old English word *boeccure* (meaning "baker").

Baldwin is a male given name, a compound of the two Germanic words, *bold* (meaning "bold or brave") and *wine* (meaning "friend").

Barack is a male given name of Arabic, Hebrew, Swahili origin meaning "thunderbolt, lightning; or blessing".

Barnett is a male given name, derived from the Old English *baernet* (literally meaning "a person who lived where land had been cleared by fire").

Barrington is a male given name of Old English origin meaning "tribe" or "settlement".

Barris is a male given name of Welsh origin meaning "son of Barry".

Barwick is a male given name of Old English origin, it is actually a locational name or place name for people coming from an outlying corn farm (from *bere* (meaning "barley or corn") and *wic* (meaning "an outlying farm").

Basil is a given name that comes from the male Greek name *Vassilios*, which first appeared during the Hellenistic period. It is derived from *basileus* (a Greek word of pre-Hellenic origin meaning "king"), from which words such as *basilica* and *basilisk* (via Latin) as well as the eponymous herb (via Old French) derive, and the name of the Italian region *Basilicata*, which had been long under the rule of the Byzantine Emperor (also called *basileus*). This name was brought to England by the Crusaders, having been common in the eastern Mediterranean. It is more often used in Britain and Europe than in the US and is also the name of a common herb. In Arabic, Basil is a name for boys that means "brave, fearless, and intrepid."

Bellamy is a male given name derived from the Old French *bel amy* (fair friend, beautiful friend), which is from the Latin *bellus* (fair, beautiful) and *amicus* (friend).

Benedict (BEN-a-dikt) is a given name, which comes from

Late Latin word *Benedictus* (meaning "blessed"). Etymologically, it is derived from the Latin words *bene* (good) + *dicte* (speak) i.e. "well spoken." The name was borne by Saint Benedict of Nursia, the founder of the Order of Saint Benedict and thereby of Western Monasticism. This name was also borne by the American general Benedict Arnold (1741-1801), who defected to Britain during the American Revolution. Shakespeare's Benedick in "Much Ado about Nothing" is a self-assured, witty bachelor.

Bennett is a male given name of English origin meaning "blessed".

Blaine is a male given name of Gaelic origin meaning "yellow".

Blake is a male given name of Old English origin meaning "dark".

Bodhi is a Hindu name, from the Sanskrit *Bodhi* (meaning "awakened, enlightened"). In Buddhist philosophy, the path to liberation from the cycle of rebirth (*moksha*) is a path of coming out of delusional beliefs to find the Truth. This path is referred to as the awakening, which results in an understanding of life and consciousness - or *bodhi*. Some individuals who reach this spiritual understanding may enter into the state of *bodhicitta*, where they assist and serve others on the path to enlightenment.

In some schools of Buddhism, it is thought that bodhi is inherent in the mind and that individuals must remove distractions in order to obtain or behold it. Yogacara Buddhism, a school of Buddhism that centers on seeing the world through the practice of yoga, also holds this belief.

Bowie is a rarely used male given name that means "yellow or fair-haired." Usage of the name is likely in reference to legendary English musician *David Bowie*.

Bradshaw is male given name that derived from two Old English words, *brade* (meaning "broad") and *sceaga* (meaning "a thicket").

Bryden is a male given name of Celtic origin meaning "a hill".

Burnett is a male given name of Old French origin meaning "brunette".

Burton is a male given name of Old English origin meaning "a settlement" or "fort".

Byron is a male given name derived from the Old English surname *aet thaem byrum*, which literally translates into "at the barns or cowsheds".

Caelum is a rare male given name meaning "heaven".

Cain is a male given name of Hebrew origin meaning "brought in". Cain was the son of Adam and Eve in the Bible and killed his brother Abel out of jealousy.

Cale is a male given name, a short form of *Caleb*.

Caleb (KAY-leb) is an ancient Hebrew name that first appears in the Old Testament's Book of Exodus (Caleb was a contemporary of Moses). The name comes from the Hebrew *Kalebh* (meaning, quite literally, "dog-like"). Caleb was one of two (Joshua being the other) who set out with Moses from Egypt and lived long enough to reach the Promised Land (Numbers 26:65). As an English name, Caleb came into use after the Protestant Reformation. It was common among the Puritans, who introduced it to America in the 17th century.

Campbell is a male given name of Gaelic origin derived from the Gaelic words *cam* (meaning "crooked or winding") and *beul* (meaning "mouth").

Carl is a male given name, a German variant of Charles, meaning "free man".

Casper is a male given name, a Dutch and Scandinavian variant of *Jasper*. Jasper originates in Persian language and means "king of the treasure".

Caspian is a given name that comes from the city of *Qazvin* (Kasbin), which was named after the *Cas* (a tribe that lived south of the Caspian Sea). In addition, Caspian is one of the main characters (a prince, and later king) in "The Chronicles of Narnia", a series of seven fantasy novels for children.

Cedric is a male given name of Old Welsh origin, derived from a combination of words *ced* (meaning "bounty") and *drych* (meaning "pattern"). Hence, the meaning is "person with generous and friendly traits".

Chandler is a male given name of French origin meaning "candle maker".

Channing (CHAN-een) is both a surname and a given name of English and Old French origin meaning "young wolf; wolf cub."

Chauncy is a male given name meaning "gamble, fortune".

Chester is a male given name of Latin origin meaning "fortress, walled town".

Chord is a very unique male given name. In music, it means aggregate of musical pitches sounded simultaneously; in geometry, a line segment joining two points on a curve.

Christopher (KRIS-toh-fer) is a given name that comes from the Greek *Khristophoros* (*Khristos* (Christ) + *pherein* (to bear)). Christopher essentially means "bearer of Christ." The name was always popular among early Christians who literally translated the name to mean "bearing Christ in their hearts." As an English given name, Christopher has been in general use since the 15th century. In Denmark, it was borne by three kings (their names are usually spelled *Christoffer*), including the 15th-century Christopher of Bavaria who also ruled Norway and Sweden. Other famous bearers include Italian explorer

Christopher Columbus (1451-1506).

Clark is a male given name, derived from the Old English term *clerk*, used to describe any member of a religious order.

Colson is a male given name, a derivative of *Nicholas*. Nicholas originates in Greek language and means "people's triumph". Other variation of Nicholas is male name *Claus*.

Conan is a boy's name of Celtic origin meaning "little wolf; little hound." It might also derive from *conn* (wisdom, counsel, strength).

Cornelius (kor-NEEL-yus) is an originally Roman masculine name. Its derivation is uncertain but is suspected to be from the Latin *cornu* that means "horn." In Acts in the New Testament Cornelius is a centurion who is directed by an angel to seek Peter. After speaking with Peter he converts to Christianity, and he is traditionally deemed the first gentile convert. The name was also borne by a few early saints, including a 3rd-century pope. In England, it came into use in the 16th century, partly due to Dutch influence.

Coven is a male given name, from Latin *conventum* (convention). The word "coven" (that usually refers to a group or gathering of witches) remained largely unused in English until 1921 when Margaret Murray promoted the idea that all witches across Europe met in groups of thirteen which they called "covens."

Crawford is a male given name of English origin that literally means "crow ford".

Cullen is the transferred use of an Irish surname from the ancient Gaelic name *Cuileannain*, which means "son of the holy one" (*cuileann* (holy) + *ain* (son)).

Cyrus (SY-russ) is the anglicized form of the Greek name *Kyros* (meaning "lord").

The name was borne by several kings of Persia, but most notably *Cyrus the Great* who reigned over the largest empire the world had yet seen (6th century B.C.). Cyrus the Great is also a prominent and admired figure in the Old Testament, noted for overthrowing the Babylonian Empire and, in an act of diplomatic genius, invited the Jews back from exile to rebuild their Temple in Jerusalem (Ezra 1:2-4). This edict made him extremely popular in the ancient Near East and he is mentioned several times in the Bible as well as the Hidden Books of the Apocrypha. As an English name, Cyrus was adopted by the Puritans during the 16th century Protestant Reformation, probably in a nod to Cyrus' appreciation for religious freedom and tolerance.

Dallas is a male given name of Scottish origin meaning "living on a clearing".

Dalton is a male given name of Old English origin meaning "settlement or village".

Damian (DAY-mee-en) is a given name that means "to tame, subdue", though the Greek root is also close to the word for "spirit." The Belgian priest Father Damien is honored as the man who helped the lepers of Molokai in Hawaii. Saint Damian was martyred with his twin brother Cosmo in

Syria early in the 4th century. They are the patron saints of physicians. Due to his renown, the name came into general use in Christian Europe. Another saint by this name was Peter Damian, an 11th-century cardinal, and theologian from Italy.

Damon is a given name derived from Greek *damazo* (means "to tame"). The Greek mythological tale of Damon and Pythias, symbolizing the loyal bonds of friendship, is said to have taken place 2,400 years ago in ancient Syracuse (modern-day Sicily). According to legend, the very paranoid ruler Dionysius the Elder believed Pythias was plotting against him and so he sentenced the young man to death. Pythias asked for a brief pardon so that he could put his affairs in order prior to his execution. Dionysius refused, but finally agreed to allow Damon, Pythias' friend, to replace him in the condemned jail cell and risk his own head should Pythias not return as promised. Pythias did return to spare his friend in the nick of time and face his own death (after a dramatic delay that included a pirated ship and a long swim back). Damon had never doubted his friend's return. Dionysius was so impressed by the trust and friendship between the two men, he released them both. Damon is, therefore, a model of loyal friendship and trust in Greek mythology. As an English given name, it has only been regularly used since the 20th century.

Dante (DAHN-tay) is a contracted form of the Italian name *Durante*, which means "steadfast, enduring" from the Latin *durus* (meaning "hard, firm"). The name Dante was most famously borne by Dante Alighieri, the 13th-century poet who gave the world one of the greatest pieces of literature in the Middle Ages, "The Divine Comedy."

Darko is a common South Slavic masculine given name. It is derived from the Slavic root *dar* (gift). Its oldest mention is from the 14th century, included in the Decani chrysobulls (1330).

Dayron is a Modern English name with no known meaning. Dayron may be a variant spelling of the name *Darren*, but its historical usage suggests otherwise. While most acknowledged respellings of Darren experienced their peak in the late 1960s and early 1970s, Dayron did not reach its peak in popularity until the early 2000s. It is therefore likely that Dayron was conceived independently of *Darren*.

Dean is a male given name, derived from the Old English word *denu* (meaning "valley") and is a locational name denoting that the bearer resided in a valley.

Denver is a male given name, derived from the Old English phrase *dena faer* (meaning "the passage of Danes").

Derek is a male given name of German origin meaning "the people's ruler."

Dexter is a male given name, derived from the Old English word *deag* (meaning "dye"). It is an occupational name, denoting that the bearer is of a certain occupation, in this case the dyeing of cloth.

Dominic is a male given name of Latin origin meaning "Lord's child".

Dorian is a male given name of Greek origin. In Greek, the name refers to either *Doris* (a district of Greece), or *Doros* (a legendary Greek hero). Doros was the son of Hellen of Sparta (who was the daughter of Zeus and Leda) and the founder of the Dorian tribe (an obscure, ancient Hellenic tribe that were supposed to have existed in the north-eastern regions of Greece, ancient Macedonia and Epirus). The most likely origin of Doros' name is the Greek word *doron* (means "gift"). Another possible origin of this name is from the

Greek *dorios* (means "child of the sea").

Also, Dorian Gray is the subject of a full-length portrait in oil by Basil Hallward, in Oscar Wilde's famous philosophical novel "The Picture of Dorian Gray."

Blinded by his youth and beauty, Dorian expresses the desire to sell his soul, to ensure that the picture, rather than he, will age and fade. The wish is granted, and Dorian pursues a libertine life of varied amoral experiences while staying young and beautiful; all the while, his portrait ages and records every his sin.

Drake is a male given name of English origin meaning "dragon".

Draven is a name taken from a 1994 action film called "The Crow." Eric Draven is resurrected from the death and spends the course of the movie avenging the brutal death of his girlfriend. Draven quite obviously is a play on words (D'Raven). Aside from the name's connection to "The Crow", Draven is an actual Anglo-Saxon surname derived from the Old English word *draefend* (meaning "hunter").

Dwight is a male given name of German origin meaning "white or blond". It is also a variation of name *Dionysos*, a Greek mythology god of grape harvest, winemaking and wine.

Edgar is a given name derived from the Old English *Eadgar* (*ēad* (prosperity, fortune, riches) + *gar* (a spear): hence, "spear of prosperity"). This name historically associated with the tenth-century English king known as *Edgar the Peaceful.* It was considered a peaceful reign due to the lack of Viking invasions or other foreign raids during his time in power. He was also successful in politically uniting the various kingdoms throughout England under one throne. There was also King *Edgar of Scotland.*

Edison (ED-ih-sun) is the transferred use of an Old English patronymic surname derived from the ancient personal name *Eadwig* (and so means "son of Eadwig"). Others conjecture that Edison might also be a variation of *Addison*, which also developed as a patronymic surname meaning "son of Adam" (Adam being the Hebrew word for "earth"). *Addie* was a common Scottish Lowlands nickname for *Adam*, and because Edison sounds a lot like *Addison* it may just represent a slight dialectal difference. In any case, the surname Edison is most commonly associated with prolific American inventor Thomas Edison (1847-1931) known mainly as the inventor of the light bulb.

Edmund is one of the oldest Anglo-Saxon names, composed of the Old English elements *ead* (wealth, fortune) and *mund* (protection). This was the name of two Anglo-Saxon kings of England. It was also borne by two saints, including a 9th-century king of East Anglia who, according to tradition, was shot to death with arrows after refusing to divide his Christian kingdom with an invading pagan Danish leader. This Old English name remained in use after the Norman conquest (even being used by King Henry III for one of his sons), though it became less common after the 15th century.

Egbert is a given name of Old English origin that means "brilliant sword" (*edge* (sword) + *beorht* (bright, famous)).

Einar is a given name derived from the Old Norse name *Einarr* (means "one warrior"). Name Einar is directly connected with the concept of the *einherjar* (warriors who died in battle and ascended to Valhalla in Norse mythology).

Elijah (ee-LYE-jah) is a male given name that comes from the Bible. Elijah was a Hebrew prophet and miracle worker, as told in the two Books of Kings in the Old Testament. Fittingly, the name Elijah comes from the Hebrew meaning "Yahweh is God" or "Jehovah is Lord." He was active in the 9th century BC during the reign of King Ahab of Israel and his Phoenician-born queen Jezebel. Elijah confronted the king and queen over their idolatry of the Canaanite god Ba'al and other wicked deeds. At the end of his life, he was carried to heaven in a chariot of fire and was succeeded by Elisha. According to Jewish tradition, Elijah is still roaming the earth and will appear when it comes time to announce the Messiah.

Elon is a male name of Hebrew origin meaning "oak tree".

Emerson (EH-mer-suhn) is a boy's name of German origin meaning "son of Emery." Emerson is a dignified, somewhat serious name associated with transcendental thinker Ralph Waldo Emerson. George Emerson, the principal male character in E. M. Forster's 1908 novel, "A Room with a View," is another literary namesake. Nowadays, ranks highly as a girl's name.

Emmet (EHM-it) is a boy's name of Hebrew origin meaning "universal; truth." Transferred use of the surname, itself derived from a diminutive of the medieval female given name Emma. Also possibly derived from Old German meaning "energetic, powerful", or from Old English meaning "an ant." The name is given to boys as a mark of respect to the great Irish orator and patriot Robert Emmet who was a leader of the unsuccessful 1798 rebellion against the British. He was captured on August 25, 1803, and tried for high treason and sentenced to be hanged, drawn and quartered. When asked if he had anything to say in response to this sentence Emmet gave what is considered to be one of the most moving speeches of the period: "When my country takes her place among the nations of the earth, then, and not till then, let my epitaph be written. I have done."

Emilian is a male given name, which comes from the Latin *Aemilius*, an old Roman family name probably derived from *aemulus* (rival, laborious, and eager).

Enver is both a masculine given name and a surname. In Turkish, Albanian and Bosnian, it is the transliteration of the Arabic name *Anwar*, which means "luminous".

Enzo is an Italian given name. The Italian and French name Enzo has three possible etymologies. In Italy, the name could have originated as an Old Italian form of the German *Heinz*, a pet form of *Heinrich* (the old German masculine name which gave the English *Henry*). From this perspective, Enzo would mean "ruler of the home" (*heim* (home) + *rīc* (power, rule)). Secondly, both the French and the Italians could have developed Enzo from another ancient German name *Anzo* (meaning (ironically) "the giant"). More modern beliefs suggest Enzo is simply a short form of Italian names like *Lorenzo* and *Vincenzo*. Enzo was the name of a king of Sardinia in the 13th century and Enzo Ferrari was the founder of the Ferrari motor company.

Eric (AIR-ik) is a male given name derived from the Old Norse *Eiríkr* (*ei* (ever, always) + *ríkr* (ruler)). Scandinavian legend relates that the explorer *Leif Ericson* (son of Erik the Red, the founder of the first Norse settlement in Greenland and Thjodhild, both of Norwegian origin) landed on the shores of America nearly four centuries years before Christopher Columbus arrived in 1492. Around A.D. 1000, Eriksson sailed to Norway, where King Olaf I converted him to Christianity. According to one school of thought, Eriksson sailed off course on his way back to Greenland and landed on the North American continent, where he explored a region he called *Vinland.* He may also have sought out Vinland based on stories of an earlier voyage by an Icelandic trader. After spending the winter in Vinland, Leif sailed back to Greenland, and never returned to North American shores. He is generally believed to be the first European to reach the North American continent.

This common Norse name was first brought to England by Danish settlers during the Anglo-Saxon period. It was not popular in England in the Middle Ages, but it was revived in the 19th century, in part due to the children's novel "Eric, or Little by Little" (1858) by Frederic William Farrar.

Erling is a male given name of Old Norse origin meaning "nobleman's offspring".

Everett is a male given name of botn Old English and Old Germanic origin meaning "wild boar".

Ezra is a male given name of Hebrew origin meaning "help".

Faust is a male given name of Latin origin meaning "fortunate".

Ferit is a male given name of Turkish origin meaning "unparalleled".

Finch is a boy's name of English origin. The ancestors of the Finch family lived among the ancient Anglo-Saxon tribes of Britain. Finch was a name given to a person who was referred to as a finch deriving from the small songbird's name. The surname may have also an occupational origin, denoting someone who caught and sold finches. Finch was also the surname of the Earls of Winchilsea and Nottingham (now Finch-Hatton) and Earls of Aylesford (now Finch-Knightley).

Finley is male given name of Scottish origin, from the Gaelic personal name *Fionnlagh* (composed of the elements *fionn* (meaning "white", "fair") + *laoch* (meaning "warrior", "hero").

Fitzgerald is a male given name of Norman origin meaning "the son of Gerald".

Frederick (FRED-er-ik) is an English form of a Germanic name meaning "peaceful ruler" (derived from *frid* (peace) + *ric* (ruler, power)). This name has long been common in continental Germanic-speaking regions, being borne by rulers of the Holy Roman Empire, Germany, Austria, Scandinavia, and Prussia. Notables among these rulers include the 12th-century Holy Roman Emperor and crusader *Frederick I Barbarossa*, the 13th-century emperor and patron of the arts *Frederick II*, and the 18th-century Frederick II of Prussia, known as *Frederick the Great.*

Gabriel is a given name that means "God is my strength." Gabriel is an archangel in Hebrew tradition, often appearing as a messenger of God. Gabriel is mentioned in the Bible once in the Old Testament and once in the New. In the Old Testament, he appears to the prophet Daniel, delivering explanations of Daniel's visions (Daniel 8:15–26, 9:21–27). In the Gospel of Luke, Gabriel appears to the Virgin Mary and to Zechariah, foretelling the births of Jesus and John the Baptist, respectively (Luke 1:11–38). The feast day of the Archangel Gabriel is traditionally celebrated by the Catholic Church on September 29 and by the Orthodox Church on November 8. A female version of the name is *Gabriela* (or *Gabriella*). Girls who are named Gabriella often take on a shorter version of the name, such as *Bella*, *Ella*, *Gabbi*, *Gabby*, *Gabi*, *Gabie*, *Gabbie* or *Gaby*.

Gannicus is a male given name that associates with a Celtic slave, who became one of the leaders of the rebel slaves during the Third Servile War (73-71 BC).

Gannon (GAN-on) is a male name of Irish and Gaelic origin meaning "fair-skinned, fair-haired".

Garrett is a male given name of Germanic origin meaning "hardy".

Gaspard is a male given name, derives from a Persian word *kaspur*, which means "treasurer." The title was given to one of the three wise men who brought gifts to the birth of Christ.

Gerald (JARE-ald) is a masculine German given name meaning "rule of the spear" (from the prefix *ger* (spear) and suffix *wald* (rule)). There were various medieval saints who bore the name Gerald, including the 9th century *Gerald of Aurillac*, a French nobleman who gave up his possessions in order to live his life in the name of Christ. Due to his childhood illness, his adult blindness and his apparent disfigurement from acne, St. Gerald of Aurillac became a patron saint to the disabled and handicapped. Gerald in England dropped from usage in the later Middle Ages until experiencing a revival in the 19th century (thanks, in part, to the influence of the Irish who never lost interest in this name). The 38th President of the United States, *Gerald Ford*, is one of the most famous name bearers in more modern times. Variants include the English given name *Jerrold*, and the feminine nickname *Jeri*.

Gerard is a male given name of Germanic origin meaning "strong like a spear".

Gibson is a male given name of Old English origin meaning "bright" or "noble".

Gilbert (GIL-bert) is a masculine name rooted in the ancient Frankish-Germanic elements *gisil* (pledge, hostage) and *berth* (bright, famous). The name was introduced to England by the Normans where it was popular during the Middle Ages. *St. Gilbert of Sempringham* used his inherited wealth to found the

Gilbertines, a religious order which included both priests and nuns (he is noted as the only Englishman to have done so). Eventually, his order would be disbanded when King Henry VIII cut ties with Rome, replaced Catholicism with the Church of England and suppressed all the monasteries. St. Gilbert is still celebrated on his Feast Day of February 4th. The name Gilbert was mainly bestowed in his honor during the Middle Ages but gained wider appeal in the 19th century.

Godfrey is a male given name, derived from Old Germanic words *guda* (meaning "good") and *frid* (meaning "peace").

Grayson is the transferred use of an English surname derived from an occupational name. The name originates from the Middle English *greyve*, which came from the Old Norse-Viking *greifi* and signifies a person holding the position of a steward (someone in charge of an estate or property). The words actually mean "count" or "earl" since the steward was high-ranking and appointed by the monarchy to oversee/govern specific land or property. The name Grayson basically indicated the son of a steward.

Griffin is a male given name of Old Welsh origin meaning "fierce person".

Gunther is a male given name of Anglo-Saxon origin meaning "battle-army".

Gustav (GOO-stahv) is a male given name of likely Old Swedish origin used mainly in Sweden, Norway, Denmark, Finland, Iceland, Estonia, France, Germany, Austria, the Netherlands, Belgium, Switzerland, and South Africa, possibly meaning "staff of the Geats or Goths or gods", possibly derived from the Old Norse elements *Gautr* (Geats), *Gutar/Gotar* (Goths), *goð ōs* (gods) and the word *stafr* (staff). Another etymology speculates that the name may be of Medieval Slavic origin, from the name *Gostislav*, a compound word for "glorious guest", from the Medieval Slavic words *Gosti* (guest) and *slava* (glory) and was adopted by migrating groups north and west into Germany and Scandinavia. This name has been borne by eight Kings of Sweden, including the 16th-century *Gustav Vasa* and the current king, *Carl XVI Gustaf.* It is a common name for Swedish monarchs since the reign of Gustav Vasa.

Hamilton is a noble male given name of Old English origin, derived from the words *hamel* (meaning "bare") and *dun* (meaning "hill").

Harris is a male given name of Germanic origin meaning "ruler of the house".

Hartwell is a unique male given name of Old English origin.

Hector (HEK-tor) is an English, French, Scottish, and Spanish given name. In Greek legend, Hector was one of the Trojan champions who fought against the Greeks. After he killed Achilles' friend Patroclus in battle, he was himself brutally slain by Achilles, who proceeded to tie his dead body to a chariot and drag it about. This name also appears in Arthurian legends belonging to King Arthur's foster father.

The name *Hektor* is probably derived from the Greek *ekhein*, meaning "to check", "restrain."

Hugh is a male given name of German, English, Irish origin meaning "mind, intellect".

Hugo is a male given name of Germanic origin, meaning "mind". The name is one of the most popular throughout Europe, also ranking among the top 10 in Spain and Belgium in the last decade.

Isaiah is a male given name of Hebrew origin, derived from two words, *yahweh* (meaning "God"), and *sha* (meaning "to deliver").

Ivar is a given name introduced by Scandinavian settlers. It is derived from the Old Norse elements *yŕ* (yew, bow) and *herr* (warrior, army): hence, "archer, bow warrior."

Jacob is a male given name of Hebrew origin meaning "following after".

Jagger is a male given name that developed from an occupation name during the Middle Ages but especially Yorkshire dialect where the Middle English word *jag* (meaning "pack, load") was used in reference to a *jagger* - i.e., a peddler or hawker of goods. Kind of like a modern-day door-to-door salesman.

The first recorded spelling of this surname appeared in Yorkshire in the late 14th century (rendered as "Jager"). Because Jagger was an occupation name turned surname so connected to Yorkshire, it is believed most modern-day Jaggers are ultimately descended from this medieval family of "peddlers." The rise in popularity of the name is likely due to the popularity of English rock star *Mick Jagger* (the lead vocalist and founding member of the legendary rock and roll band "the Rolling Stones").

Jamison literally means "son of James" (though originally a surname from Scotland and

Ireland, Jamison is also used as a first name by parents who fear the name "James Jr.").

Jasper is a male given name of Persian origin meaning "bringer of treasure".

Jenkins is a male given name of Hebrew origin meaning "God is merciful".

Jeremiah is a male given name of Hebrew origin meaning "lifted up by God".

Joris is a male given name derived from the Greek *geōrgos* (earth-worker, farmer), which is composed of the elements *gē* (earth) and *ergein* (to work).

Julian (JOO-lee-ən or JOOL-yən) is a male given name derived from the Latin *Iulus* (the first down on the chin, downy-bearded). Because a person just beginning to develop facial hair is young, "youth" became an accepted meaning of the name. This was the name of the last pagan Roman emperor, Julian the Apostate (4th century). It was also borne by several early saints, including the legendary Saint Julian the Hospitaller. This name has been used in England since the Middle Ages, at which time it was also a feminine name (from *Juliana*, eventually becoming *Gillian*).

Kai is a male given name originated from several possible sources: might be a variation of the Latin name *Gaius* or the short form of *Kylie*; also means "sea water" in Hawaiian.

Kaj is a male given name of Danish origin meaning "Earth".

Keanu is a male given name of Hawiian origin meaning "cool breeze".

Kellen (KEL-en) is a rarely used name of Gaelic origin that can mean "slender" or "thin."

Kenneth (KEN-eth) is an English given name and surname. This name is an Anglicised form of two entirely different Gaelic personal names: *Cainnech* and *Cináed*. The modern Gaelic form of *Cainnech* is *Coinneach*; the name was derived from a byname meaning "handsome" or "comely." The name *Cinaed* is partly derived from the Celtic *aidhu* (meaning "fire"). This name was borne by the Scottish king *Kenneth* (*Cináed*) *mac Alpin*, who united the Scots and Picts in the 9th century. It was popularized outside of Scotland by Sir Walter Scott, who used it for the hero in his novel "The Talisman" (1825). A famous bearer was the British novelist *Kenneth Grahame* (1859-1932), who wrote "The Wind in the Willows."

Kylian (KIL-ee-an) is a given name of Celtic-Gaelic origin that means "war and strife".

Lawford is a male given name of English origin meaning "from a ford on the hill".

Leon (LAY-on) is a first name of Greek origin that means "lion." Perhaps the oldest attested historical figure to bear this name was *Leon of Sparta*, a 5th-century BCE king of Sparta, while in Greek mythology Leon was a Giant killed by Heracles. During the Christian era, Leon was merged with the Latin cognate *Leo*, with the result that the two forms are used interchangeably. A similar Greek name to Leon is *Leonidas* (meaning "son of a lion"), with *Leonidas I*, king of Sparta, being perhaps the most famous bearer of that name.

Levon (LEE-von) is an Armenian given name, equivalent to *Leon*. This was the name of several kings of Cilician Armenia, including the first king *Levon I the Magnificent*.

Lockwood is a male given name of Old English origin meaning "a wood encircled by a fence".

Louis is a French name that ultimately derived from the Old German *Chlodowig*, and means "famous in battle" or "famous warrior".

Lucas is a male given name that means "man from Lucania", referring to the southern region of Italy. The region was so-named to translate to "bright" or "shining". Closely related to the names Lucio and Luke, the popularity of Lucas can also be attributed to Saint Luke the Evangelist, considered to be the inspiration for the name's popularity in the Middle Ages.

Luchie is a very extraordinary and unusual name. There is no information about its origin and meaning; the only thing we know is that the name *Luchie* is ranked on the 20000 position of the most used names. It means that this name is very rarely used.

Lucian (LOO-shun) is a sleeker, more sophisticated version of *Lucius* (LOO-sias). It is a first name of Latin origin that means "light."

The name Lucius predates Christ by several centuries and was held by a couple of early Etruscan kings of ancient Rome as well as several other prominent Romans of Antiquity. Lucius was also borne by three Popes and several early saints. The name is mentioned briefly in the New Testament in reference to *Lucius of Cyrene* who established the Christian Church in Antioch. Despite the name's Christian connections, it never became a heavily used or wide-spread name in medieval Europe. It wasn't until the

Renaissance (14th to 17th centuries) that Lucius got noticed.

Ludwig is a male given name of German origin meaning "famous warrior".

Magnus (MAG-ness), meaning "great" in Latin, was sometimes used as a first name among Romans but was not particularly common among them. The best-known Roman bearing the name was the third-century usurper. The name gained wider popularity in the Middle Ages, among various European peoples and their royal houses, being introduced to them upon being converted to the Latin-speaking Catholic Christianity.

This was especially the case with Scandinavian royalty and nobility.

Malcolm is a Scottish male given name, an Anglicized form of the Old Gaelic name *Mael Coluimb*, meaning "devotee of Saint Columba".

Marcel (mar-SELL) is an Occitan form of the Ancient Roman origin male given name *Marcellus*, meaning "belonging to Mars."

Marco is an Italian masculine given name of Latin origin. The name is common in Italy, Austria, Portugal, the Netherlands, and Switzerland.

It derives from the ancient Latin god *Mars*.

Marcus (MAR-kus) is a masculine given name of Ancient Roman pre-Christian origin derived either from Etruscan *Marce* of unknown meaning (possibly from the Etruscan *mar* (to harvest)), or referring to the god *Mars* (god of War).

Marley, as a given name, comes from a surname which was taken from a place name meaning either "pleasant wood", "boundary wood", or "marten wood" in Old English. A famous bearer of the surname was the Jamaican musician Bob Marley (1945-1981).

Mateo is a male given name of Spanish, Italian, Latin origin meaning "gift of God".

Matthias is a male given name, a variant of *Matthew*, meaning "God's present".

Maurice is a French male given name deriving from the Latin *Mauritius*. Mauritius was a saint, and the name was used in the Roman Empire period, referring to "one from Mauritania" (or "the Moor").

Maverick (MA-və-rik) is a boy's name of American origin meaning "independent, nonconformist."

Maximilian is a given name that comes from the Latin *Maximilianus* (greatest). Maximilian became a traditional name among the royal Habsburg family members in Austria-Hungary as well as the royal house of Bavaria.

Milo (MIE-lo) is a masculine given name and a surname, Old Germanic form of *Miles*, derived from the Latin word for "soldier." Alternatively, it might be from the Old Slavonic root *milu* (merciful).

Murphy is an Irish male given name, derived from the Celtic name *O'Murchadha* (meaning "descendant of Murchadh"). The name *Murchadh* itself is derived from the word *muir* (meaning "the sea").

Myron is a masculine given name used in English-speaking and Eastern European countries, including Romania, Ukraine, and Russia (in the former USSR it is usually spelled *Miron*); this name derived from Greek *myron* (meaning "sweet oil, perfume").

Nathan is a male given name derived from the Hebrew verb *gave*, Nathan originated from the Hebrew name Natan, Yiddish Nussen or Tiberian Hebrew Natan. It may translate to "he has given" or "he will give".

Nelson is a male given name of Gaelic origin meaning "coming from clouds".

Nero is a male given name of Latin origin meaning "the strong one".

Nolan is an Irish name originating from the transferred use of a surname *Ó Nualláin* (meaning "a descendant of Nuallán"). The Gaelic *nuall* means "chariot-fighter, champion."

Norris is a male given name of Old French origin meaning "coming from North".

Norwood is a male given name that comes from a surname,

which was originally taken from a place name meaning "north wood" in Old English.

Orlando is a male given name of Italian origin meaning "famous throughout the land".

Osborn is a male given name of Old English origin meaning "god of bears".

Oscar is a male given name of Gaelic origin meaning "friend of the deer".

Oswald (OZ-wald) is a masculine given name derived from the Old English elements *os* (god) and *weald* (power, ruler). Saint Oswald was a king of Northumbria who introduced

Christianity to northeast England in the 7th century before being killed in battle. There was also an Old Norse cognate Ásvaldr in use in England, being borne by the 10th-century Saint Oswald of Worcester, who was of Danish ancestry. Though the name had died out by the end of the Middle Ages, it was revived in the 19th century.

Paolo (PA-o-lo) is both a given name and a surname, the Italian form of the name *Paul* (from the Latin *Paulus*, which originated as a Roman family name derived from *paulus* (small)). Paul was the adopted name of *Saul of Tarsus*, a Jewish Roman citizen converted to Christianity by a vision of Christ which blinded him for several days. He became one of the great missionary apostles and authored several New Testament epistles.

Pascal is a common boys name in France, Pascal translates as Pasquale in Italian, Pascual in Spanish and Pasqual in Catalan. The name has origins in the Latin word *paschalis* (meaning "relating to Easter").

Patrocle is a given name derived from the Ancient Greek name *Pátroklos* (*patrós* (father) + *kléos* (good report, fame, and glory)). In turn, the name means "glory of the father." In Greek mythology, Patroklos was the son of Menoetius, grandson of

Actor, King of Opus, and was Achilles' beloved comrade and brother-in-arms. From the same elements, arranged in reverse order, is also formed the name Cleopatra.

Pearson is a male given name, ultimately derived from name *Peter*, meaning "rock".

Perseus is a male given name derived from Greek *pertho* (meaning "to destroy").
In Greek mythology, Perseus was the slayer of the Gorgon Medusa and the rescuer of *Andromeda* from a sea monster. He was the son of Zeus and Danaë, the daughter of Acrisius of Argos. As an infant Perseus was cast into the sea in a chest

with his mother by Acrisius, to whom it had been prophesied that he would be killed by his grandson. After Perseus had grown up on the island of Seriphus, where the chest had grounded, King Polydectes of Seriphus, who desired Danaë, tricked Perseus into promising to obtain the head of Medusa, the only mortal among the Gorgons.

Aided by Hermes and Athena, Perseus pressed the Graiae, sisters of the Gorgons, into helping him by seizing the one eye and one tooth that the sisters shared and not returning them until they provided him with winged sandals (which enabled him to fly), the cap of

Hades (which conferred invisibility), a curved sword, or sickle, to decapitate Medusa, and a bag in which to conceal the head. (According to another version, the Graiae merely directed him to the Stygian Nymphs, who told him where to find the Gorgons and gave him the bag, sandals, and helmet; Hermes gave him the sword.) Because the gaze of Medusa turned all who looked at her to stone, Perseus guided himself by her reflection in a shield given him by Athena and beheaded Medusa as she slept. He then returned to Seriphus and rescued his mother by turning Polydectes and his supporters to stone at the sight of Medusa's head.

A further deed attributed to Perseus was his rescue of the Ethiopian princess Andromeda when he was on his way home with Medusa's head. Andromeda's mother, Cassiopeia, had claimed to be more beautiful than the sea nymphs, or Nereids; so Poseidon had punished Ethiopia by flooding it and plaguing it with a sea monster.
An oracle informed Andromeda's father, King Cepheus, that the ills would cease if he exposed Andromeda to the monster, which he did. Perseus, passing by, saw the princess and fell in love with her. He turned the sea monster to stone by showing it Medusa's

head and afterward married Andromeda.

Later Perseus gave the Gorgon's head to Athena, who placed it on her shield, and gave his other accoutrements to Hermes. He accompanied his mother back to her native Argos, where he accidentally struck her father, Acrisius, dead when throwing the discus, thus fulfilling the prophecy that he would kill his grandfather. He consequently left Argos and founded Mycenae as his capital, becoming the ancestor of the Perseids, including Heracles.

Philip (FIL-ip) is a given name derived from the Greek *Philippos* (*phílos* (dear, loved, loving) + *hippos* (horse)). In Ancient Greece, the ownership of horses was available only to those rich enough to afford them. Thus, "lover of horses" can also be understood as "noble." In the classical period of ancient Greece, when horses were a vital part of life, Philip was a name shared by scores of men, from army generals to philosophers, from astronomers to kings of Macedon, from statesmen to poets and from historians to Emperors. From a religious perspective, Philip the Apostle was one of Jesus' Twelve Apostles and Philip the Evangelist was an enthusiastic spreader of Christianity. Philip has been a long enduring name with illustrious examples of men throughout 2500 years of history.

Pierre (pee-AIR) is a masculine given name. It is a French form of the name *Peter* (it can also be a surname and a place name). Pierre originally means "rock" or "stone" in French.

Quentin (KWEN-tin) is an old French form of the Roman name *Quintinus*, which is derivative of the Latin *quintus* (meaning "fifth"). Quintus was a given name during Antiquity and likely bestowed upon the fifth child in terms of birth order or a child born in the fifth month of the year.

Quill is a male given name of Gaelic origin meaning "from the woods".

Quincy is a male given name of French origin meaning "estate of the fifth son".

Ragnar is a fearsome Old Norse name with a long history in Scandinavia. *Ragnar Lodbrok* (meaning "shaggy pants") was a legendary warrior whose story was told in the Viking sagas. Ragnar also recalls the name of the Norse Judgment Day, *Ragnarök*. In Norse mythology, Ragnarök is a series of events, including a great battle, foretold to lead to the death of a number of great figures (including the Gods

Odin, Thor, Týr, Freyr, Heimdallr and Loki), natural disasters and the submersion of the world in water. After these events, the world will resurface anew and fertile, the surviving and returning gods will meet and the world will be repopulated by two human survivors.

Raiden is the typical English transcription of *Raijin* (the god of the thunder and lightning in Japanese mythology). The god is generally depicted as a demon-like man who beats his drum (thus creating storms and the sound of thunder). Because of the name's similarity to popular baby names Aiden and Jayden, most people will pronounce it

RAY-den, but it's more properly RYE-den.

Raphael is a male given name of Hebrew origin that means "God has healed". While a common and beloved name in France, it is also popular in Spain, Germany, Italy and Portugal.

Reginald (REJ-a-nold) is an English masculine name developed from the Germanic *Raginald* (*ragin* (advice, counsel) + *wald* (rule)). An older cognate existed in England prior to the Norman Conquest of 1066, but the Latinized version brought to England by the French (i.e., *Reginaldus*) reinforced to the usage of this old Germanic name in its newest form: Reginald. It was quite common throughout the Middle Ages. Many of the Germanic and Celtic given names incorporated "ruler", "chief", or "warrior" type meanings due to the constant atmosphere of warring tribes and the importance of effective leadership among warriors in battle. Reginald is a great example of a "wise ruler".

Richmond is a male given name, derived from the Old French words *riche* (meaning "rich" or "splendid") and *mont* (meaning "hill"). It is a locational name and means that the person comes from places in France such as Richemont or Richemond.

Ridley is a male given name of Old English origin meaning "cleared wood".

Ripley is a male given name of Medieval English origin that literally translates into "the farm whose land cuts a strip through the forest".

Reuben (ROO-ben) is a given name that means "behold, a son" in Hebrew. In the Old Testament, Reuben is the eldest son of Jacob and Leah and the ancestor of one of the twelve tribes of Israel. Reuben was cursed by his father because he slept with Jacob's concubine Bilhah. It has been used as a Christian name in Britain since the Protestant Reformation.

Rockford is a male given name of French origin meaning "strong rock".

Roderick (RAHD-ə-rik) is a Germanic given name that means "famous power" (from the Germanic elements *hrod* (fame) and *ric* (power)). This name was in use among the Normans in the form *Rodric* but was not frequent in the medieval period. It is also an anglicized form of the personal name *Rhydderch*, originally a byname meaning "reddish brown."

Roman is a male first name. It has distant origins dating back to the Roman Empire and the Latin language. It comes from the Latin word *romanus*, which means "of Rome." In this initial sense, the title "Roman" means "a citizen of the Roman Empire", a man of Roman (or Byzantine) culture, Latin or Greek.

Ronald is a male given name, derived from Old Norse elements *regin* (meaning "advice", "decision") and *valdr* (meaning "ruler", "brightness").

Rory is a given name of Gaelic origin. Anglicized form of *Ruairí* (red, rust-colored). The name was born by Rory O'Connor, the last high king of Ireland, who reigned from 1166 - 1170. That's why the main meaning of the name is "red king."

Ryker is a male given name of German origin meaning "rich".

Sandor is a male given name, a Hungarian variant of *Alexander*, meaning "defender of man".

Sawyer is a boy's name of English origin; an occupational name for someone who earned his living by sawing wood. Popularized by the fictional young boy who persuades his friends to whitewash a fence for him in the 1876 Mark Twain novel, "The Adventures of Tom Sawyer."

Seaborn is a male given name of Anglo-Saxon origin meaning "sea warrior".

Sebastian is a given name that comes from the Greek name *Sebastianos* (meaning "from Sebastia"), which was the name of the city now known as *Sivas*, located in the central part of what is now Turkey. Despite Sebastian's origin in ancient Greece, it was the Christian Saint Sebastian who popularized the name across Europe and the Mediterranean. King Sebastian of Portugal, a crusader, continued the name's Christian influence. The name also appears in Shakespeare's "Twelfth Night" and "The Tempest."

Sigmund (SIG-mund) is a Germanic given name with roots in proto-Germanic *segaz* and *mundō*, giving a rough translation of "protection through victory." In Norse mythology, this was the name of the hero Sigurd's father, the bearer of the powerful sword Gram. A notable bearer was the Austrian psychologist *Sigmund Freud* (1856-1939), the creator of the revolutionary theory of psychoanalysis.

Stefan (stef-FAHN) is mainly the German and Scandinavian spelling of *Stephen*. Stephen's name comes from the Greek word *stephanos* (meaning "garland crown") and was notably borne by the very first Christian martyr in Roman Catholic tradition and so he was the first disciple of Jesus to receive the martyr's crown. His story is told in Acts 6:8-8:2 and it goes like this. The apostles ordained seven deacons to look after the care of widows and the poor, and of these chosen administrators, Stephen was the most famous. He was renowned for his eloquence and wisdom which successfully gained many Jesus followers. In fact, it might be said that Stephen was too successful for his own good because he ended up attracting the attention of some very bad men. They accused Stephen of blasphemy against Moses and God in front of an assembly of men which Stephen faced bravely (legend has it that his face took on the form of an angel). They then exacted the requisite ancient punishment of stoning to death. In his parting words, Stephen asked only for his enemies' salvation: "Lord, do not hold this sin against them." It turns out that Stephen's public stoning had the opposite effect the executioners had intended because many Christ followers fled Jerusalem fearing for their lives to Judea and Samaria, taking with them a belief system that had been relatively confined to Jerusalem. As the first Christian martyr, Stephen's feast day comes right after Jesus' on December 26. Like many names from the Bible, Stephen gained popularity in ancient times and on throughout the Middle Ages as people bestowed names upon their children in homage to those they revered.

Talbot is a male given name of English origin meaning "command of the valley".

Terrwyn is a male given name of Welsh origin meaning "valiant."

Thelonious is a male given name, ultimately derived from *Theodoric* (from words *thiuda* (meaning "people" or "race") and *reiks* (meaning "powerful" or "ruler")).

Theodore is a male given name of Greek origin meaning "gift of God".

Thorsteinn is a given name derived from Old Norse name *Þórstæinn* (*þónr* (thunder, Thor) + *steinn* (stone). In Norse mythology, Thor (Þónr) is a hammer-wielding God associated with thunder, lightning, storms, oak trees, strength, the protection of mankind, and also hallowing, healing, and fertility.

Thorvald is a given name derived from the Old Norse name *Þórvaldr*, which means "Thor's ruler" (from the name of the Norse god *Þórr* (Thor) combined with *valdr* (ruler)).

Tobias is a Greek version of the Hebrew biblical name *Toviyah* (meaning "The goodness of

God"). Since the Middle Ages, the name has mainly been associated with the Biblical tale "Tobias and the Angel", in which Tobias is the son of Tobit, a rich and righteous Jew who goes blind after bird droppings fall into his eyes. The archangel Raphael (disguised as a man) accompanies Tobias on a journey to retrieve money for Tobit. With the aid of the angel, Tobias returns from his travels triumphantly - a rich man with a new wife on his arm after defeating an evil demon. He also brings Tobit an ointment (fish gall bladder) which, after rubbed into his eyes, miraculously cures his blindness and restores his eyesight. As a result of Tobias' heroic deeds and the popularity of this story in medieval times, the name came into wider usage.

Tristan (TRISS-tan) is a given name of Welsh origin. From the Old French *Tristran*, which is from the Gaelic *Drystan*, a name derived from *drest* (tumult, riot). The name was borne in medieval legend by a knight who was sent to Israel by King Mark of Cornwall to bring Isolde back to be the king's bride. On the return trip, Tristan and Isolde accidentally drank a love potion intended for the king and fell in love. Tristan left to fight for King Howel of Brittany and, seriously wounded in battle, sent for Isolde. She arrived too late and died from grief next to Tristan's deathbed. The tale was the subject of many popular tragedies during the Middle Ages.

Tyrion is one of the many new names entering the lexicon thanks to George R. R. Martin, author of the "Game of Thrones" book. Tyrion's name shares its first two letters with those of his father *Tywin* and his grandfather *Tytos*. George Martin has said he saw the Tyrion character as being both the ugliest and the most intelligent person in the world, a mixed legacy for any child.

Tyson is an English male given name, derived from the Old French name *Tison* (meaning "son of Ty").

Ulrich is a male given name of Germanic origin meaning "rich" or "powerful".

Umberto is an Italian form of name *Humbert* (derived from the Germanic elements *hun* (meaning "bear-cub, warrior") and *berht* (meaning "bright, famous")).

Vermont is a male given name of French origin meaning "green mountain".

Vicente is the Portuguese and Spanish form of *Vincent*, both of which are derived from the Latin *vincens* (meaning "conquering, winning"). The name was borne by scores of early saints, the most notable of which was *Saint*

Vincent of Saragossa, who lived in the 3rd century. Saint Vincent of Saragossa was an outspoken and fearless Christian who lived during the period of Roman persecution. He was tortured for his beliefs and killed when he refused to burn the Scripture. It is said that ravens protected his corpse from vultures until his followers could recover his body, entomb him and build a shrine. He is now the patron saint of the Portugal capital, Lisbon, and also said to be the patron saint of wine-makers.

Wallace is a male given name of Celtic origin meaning "foreign" or "Celtic". The name started as a nick name given by the Normans to the minority of Celtic people in Scotland.

Walker is a male given name of Old English origin meaning "to roll". The name is a Medieval professional name for a person who trod on woolen cloth to thicken it and prepare it for using.

Walter is a male given name of German origin meaning "army ruler".

Warrick is a male given name of Old English origin meaning "strong leader who defends".

Weston is an Anglo-Saxon locational given name that means "west settlement".

Whitman is a male given name of English origin meaning "white man".

Wilder is a male given name of German origin that means "hunter."

Wilfred is a male given name of English origin, derived from the words *wil* (meaning "desire") and *fridu* (meaning "peace" or "safety").

Wyatt is a male given name derived from the medieval personal name *Wiot*, *Wyot*, *Gyot*, which derives from the Old English personal name *Wigheard* (*wig* (war) + *heard* (hardy, brave, strong)).

Xzavier (ZAY-vee-er) is a modern Americanized spelling variation of the Spanish name *Xavier*. The name Xavier comes from a Basque surname which originated as a place name, from the Basque word *Etcheberria* (meaning "the new house").

Yann (Ee-yahn) is a male given name of French and Hebrew origin that means "God is gracious."

Yukio is a male given name of Japanese origin meaning "happiness" or "good fortune".

Zackery is a male given name, English cognate of the Ecclesiastic Late Latin and Ecclesiastic Greek *Zacharias* (remembrance of the Lord), which is from the Hebrew *Zecharya*, a derivative of *zĕcharyah* (God remembers, memory).

Zander is the phonetic equivalent to *Xander*, a short form of *Alexander*. Alexander is the Latin form of the Greek name *Alexandros*. The name's meaning is interpreted from *alexein* (to defend) + *andros* (man, warrior) in a relationship or possessive form. Hence the meaning: "Defender of Men." The name is largely embodied by the well-known King of the Greek-influenced Macedon dating back to the 4th century BC: Alexander the Great. You'd be hard pressed to find a warrior more legendary than this man. The name was popularized in the post-Classical era throughout Europe as a common given name and shows up several times in the New Testament. There are over 40 Christian saints that bear the name Alexander. This is one of the oldest and most successful names in human history. As such, the name gave way to scores of variations, nicknames, and short forms. Xander is primarily used by the Dutch, while Zander is more typically American (English).

Zane is a male given name of Hebrew origin meaning "gift from God".

Zion (ZYE-on) is a male given name of Hebrew origin, meaning "highest point." Zion is a biblical term for the "promised land." For Rastafarians it means "heaven on Earth" and it is also widely associated with the drive for a Jewish homeland and with the ideals of the Mormon Church. A *zion* was a citadel that was in the center of Jerusalem, which explains why it means "highest point."

Names for Girls

Abilene is a female given name of Hebrew origin meaning "born where the grass grows".

Adah is a female given name of Hebrew origin meaning "from the beautiful scenery".

Adeline (ADD-a-line, add-a-LEEN) is the French diminutive of *Adèle*, a popular name since medieval times thanks to the 7th/ 8th century *St. Adele*. She was the daughter of the Frankish King Dagobert II who became a nun upon the death of her husband, founded a convent and was revered for her holiness, prudence, and compassion. Adèle was also the name borne by a daughter of William the Conqueror (which is how the name arrived in England in the 11th century). The name is Germanic in origin, from the word *adel* (meaning "noble"). Adeline has been used occasionally by English speakers since the 16th century.

Adelisa (ah-da-LEES-ah) is a feminine name of French origin that means "of the nobility" or "noble."

Adriana is a feminine given name derived from *Adrian*, which dates back to Antiquity. Adrian comes from the Latin word *hadrianus* (meaning "man from Hadria", an ancient city in northern Italy on the Adriatic Sea).

Afia is a female given name of African origin meaning "Friday born child".

Agata is a female given name, a Czech variant of *Agatha*. Agatha originates in Greek language and means "good-hearted".

Agneta is a female given name of Greek origin meaning "sacred, chaste".

Ahana is a female given name of Hindu origin meaning "immortal".

Aileen (eye-LEEN) is a variant spelling of *Eileen* which is the anglicized version of the Irish *Eibhlín* and Scottish *Eilidh*, both of which are Gaelic forms of the female name *Helen*. Helen originated from the Greek *Hēlēnē*, a name made famous by the beautiful Spartan queen whose abduction by Paris set in motion the mythological Trojan War. Also, it's a form of *hēlios* (a Greek word for "sun"), so Helen is thought to mean "ray or sunbeam".

Ai is a female given name of Chinese origin meaning "lovable".

Aisha is a female given name of Arabic origin meaning "one who is alive".

Alice is a female given name meaning "noble," derived from the ancient Greek word *Aletheia* means "truth" or "truthful one".

Almina is a rare feminine name of Old German origin that means "determined protector". Almina is an alternate spelling of *Elmina* (Old German) and a short form of *Wilhelmina*.

Alondra is a feminine given name. It is a short form of *Alejandra* (from the Greek word *alexein* (to defend) + *andros* (man, warrior (in a relationship or possessive form))). Hence the meaning: "defender of men or mankind." Alondra is also the Spanish word for "lark."

Alvina is a female given name with the meaning "elf friend", "amicable", "friendly", "warrior princess", and "magical being." In English, it is the feminine form of *Alvin*, which comes from either the Old English name *Ælfwine*, containing the words *ælf* (meaning "elf") and *wine* (meaning "friend"), or from the Old High German name *Adelwin* (meaning "noble friend"). Also, means "loved by everyone."

Amelia (a-MEEL-yah) is the Latinized form of the ancient Old High German female name

Amalia, from the Germanic element *amal* (meaning "to work"). People often confuse Amelia with *Aemilius*, an Old Roman family name of Latin origin (meaning "rival"), but this is incorrect. Aemilius gave us *Emily*, while Amelia had more "laborious" origins. The name became popular in England after the German House of Hanover came to the British throne in the 18th century - it was borne by daughters of George II and George III. Another famous bearer was *Amelia Earhart* (1897-1937), the first woman to make a solo flight over the Atlantic Ocean.

Anette is a variant form of name *Anna*. **Anna** is a Latin form of the Greek name *Ἄννα* and the Hebrew name *Hannah* (meaning "favor", "grace", or "beautiful"). Anna is in wide use in countries across the world as are its variants Anne, originally a French version of the name, though in use in English speaking countries for hundreds of years, and *Ann*, which was originally the English spelling. Saint Anne was traditionally the name of the mother of the Virgin Mary, which accounts for its wide use and popularity among Christians. The name has also been used for numerous saints and queens. **Anika** (AH-ne-kah) is the German, Dutch and

Danish variation of the name *Anne*.

Annabelle (*Annabel*, *Anabel*, *Annabell*, or *Anabelle*) is a female given name, a variant of *Amabel* probably influenced by *Anna*, which means "graceful" or "favour" and comes from Latin and Greek roots. Annabel also has part of the French word *Belle*, which means "beautiful." Belle is sometimes used as a given name in the English language. It can also be a contraction of the Spanish name "Ana Isabel."

Anneliese (AH-neh-lees) is a female given name of either German, Dutch, or Nordic origin that means "graced with God's bounty." It is a compound form of "Anna" and "Liese", a short form of "Elisabeth."

Arabella (AIR-a-bell-ah) is a feminine given name, alteration of *Annabella*, from the medieval *Amabel* (derived from the Latin *amabilis* (meaning "lovable")). Also, it could be a mutation from the Latin word *orabilis* meaning "susceptible to prayer" (from *orare* meaning "to pray"). The most notable Scottish bearer of this name was Lady *Arabella Stuart* (1575-1615) who was a possible successor to the English throne after Queen Elizabeth I of England. A ship named the *Arbella* brought a group of Puritan English aristocrats to the Massachusetts

Bay Colony in 1630; many socially prominent Boston families are descended from this group.

Araceli is a female given name of Spanish origin that means "altar of the sky" (*ara* "altar" and *coeli* "sky"). This is an epithet of the Virgin Mary in her role as the patron saint of Lucena, Spain.

Aria is a female name that means "air" and the melody "Aria" in Italian; in Albanian language means "from gold"; "lioness of God" in Hebrew; and "noble" in Persian. In music, an aria is a self-contained piece for one voice, with or without orchestral accompaniment, normally part of a larger work.

Ariana (ah-ree-AH-nə) is a female given name of Italian origin meaning "most holy." In Greek mythology, she was the daughter of Minos King of Crete, and his queen Pasiphae, daughter of Helios, the Sun-titan. *Arianna* and *Ariane* are the two most common variations.

Arielle is the French form of *Ariel*. Most etymological sources translate Ariel into the Hebrew word for "Lion of God" or "hero." It is also sometimes said to mean "alter hearth" which would make sense given the Biblical place name.

Ariel originated as a male given name in the Jewish community, with Ariella being a feminine form of the name. Arielle is the French variation also used among the English.

Aspen is the English vocabulary word, denoting a type of poplar tree, the aspen tree (a type of poplar familiar in the West, with heart-shaped leaves that quiver in the lightest breeze, hence its nickname, the "quaking" or "trembling" aspen).

Astrid is a female name primarily used in Scandinavia (although it is also used among the French and Germans to some degree). The name, rendered as *Ástríðr* in its ancient form, comes from the Old Nordic elements *ass* (meaning "god") and *friðr* (meaning "beautiful"). Some say the name essentially translates to "divinely beautiful" while others would say it means "beloved of the gods."

Audrey (AW-dree) is an English feminine given name. It is the Anglo-Norman form of the Anglo-Saxon name *Æðelþryð*, composed of the elements *æðel* (noble) and *þryð* (strength). The Anglo-Norman form of the name was applied to *Saint Audrey* (d. 679), also known by the historical form of her name as *Saint Æthelthryth*. In the 17th century, the name of Saint Audrey gave rise to the adjective tawdry "cheap and pretentious; cheaply adorned" (after a fair of St. Audrey where cheap lace was sold). As a consequence, use of the name declined, but it was revived in the 19th century. The popularity of the name in the United States peaked in the interbellum period, but it fell below rank 100 in popularity by 1940 and was not frequently given in the latter half of the 20th century. A famous bearer was British actress *Audrey Hepburn* (1929-1993).

Aurelia (aw-REEL-yah) is a female name that comes from the Latin *Aurelius* (from *aureus* meaning "golden"). The name began from minor early saints but was given as a name due to its meaning, and not from where it originated.

Aveline is a name that's long been an obscure cousin of more widely-used choices but may come into its own riding the tail of the name *Ava*. Aveline's roots, however, are not the same as Ava's bird-related origins but connect with the ancient Roman place name Avella, which means "filbert" or "hazelnut."

Avriella is a rarely used female name that comes from the Latin name *Avriel* (means "to open").

Aylin (iy-LEEN) is a female given name of Turkish origin meaning "to belong to the Moon."

Barbara is a female given name of Greek origin meaning "stranger, foreigner". Barbara was the name of several saints in Roman Catholic tradition, one of them being Saint Barbara, the protector against lightning and fire.

Beitris is a female given name, a Scottish variant of *Beatrix*. Beatrix originates in Latin language and means "voyager". Beatrix was the name of several saints in Christianity and it was also a popular given name within royalty.

Bernadette is a female given name of Old Enhlish origin meaning, a variant of *Bernard*, or *Bernarda* that means "as strong as a bear".

Bethany is a female given name of Old English origin meaning "from a fig house". It was probably derived from a place mentioned in the New Testament, the town where Lazarus lived.

Beverly is a female given name of Old English origin meaning "coming from the stream of beavers". It was derived from an Old English place name and until today appears as a place name on multiple occasions. As a feminine given name it might have been popularized by the name of a luxurios Los Angeles area, Beverly Hills.

Bianca (bee-AHN-kə) is a female given name of Italian origin meaning "white" (Italian cognate of "blanche").

Blaire is a transferred use of the Scottish surname derived from place-names containing the Gaelic element *blár* (plain, level field): hence, "dweller on the plain."

Brenda is a female given name of Old Norse origin meaning "sword".

Bridgette is a female given name of French origin meaning "strength" and is associated with the mythological Celtic goddess of fire and poetry.

Brooke is a female given name of Old English origin meaning "from a stream".

Bryana is a feminine form of *Brian*, which is believed to be of Celtic origin and of the meaning "strength."

Buffy is a female given name of Hebrew origin meaning, a diminutive of *Elizabeth* that means "promise of God".

Caoimhe (KEE-va) is a fairly common feminine name in Ireland, which comes from the Irish *caomh* (meaning dear or noble). It originates from the same root as the masculine name ***Caoimhín*** (pronounced KEE-veen).

Camille is female given name, a French take on the name *Camilla*. It is also thought to have been inspired by the word *camillus*, referring to a young acolyte in ancient Roman religion, and its Arabic meaning is "the perfect one".

Cara (KAR-ah, KEER-ah) is the Latin and Italian word for "dear" as in "cherished, beloved" but it is also the Irish-Gaelic word for "friend." Despite her many potential meanings, from a historical perspective, parents have used Cara with the Latin definition in mind to demonstrate their love for their "beloved" baby girls. The name dates back to the late 19th century but did not gain any significant popularity within the English speaking world until the 1950s. Cara is also sometimes considered a form of other "Car" names: *Carolina*, *Carina*, and *Carissa*, for instance.

Cariba is a rarely used feminine name of unknown origin and meaning. There is a version that this name is of Arab origin and means "pure", but it is not proven.

Carla is a female given name of German origin meaning "free woman".

Carmel (kar-MEL) is a feminine given name of Hebrew origin that means "garden, orchard."

Biblical place name: *Mount Carmel* is in Israel near the city of Haifa, and is often referred to as a type of paradise. In the 12th century, a monastery was founded in there, from which the Carmelite monastic order came about. The monastery was dedicated to the Virgin Mary and Carmel became one of the names taken from Marian titles, in this case, "Our Lady of Carmel." The name is used mainly by Roman Catholics and the form *Carmen* is more common.

Cecilia (sess-SEEL-yah) is a female given name that comes from the Latin *Caecilía*, which is the feminine form of the Old Roman family name *Caecilius* (from the Latin word *caecus*, which means "blind"). The name Cecilia was mainly popularized during the Middle Ages, in homage to the 2nd century *Saint Cecilia*. Cecilia refused to worship the Roman gods during the reign of Marcus Aurelius, and so was martyred after being tortured, suffocated and finally beheaded. She is the patron saint of music and musicians because as she lay dying she was said to be singing to God. The name became common among Christians during the Middle Ages when it was brought by the Normans to England, where it was commonly spelled *Cecily*.

Celeste is a feminine given name that derives from the Latin *caelestis* (meaning "heavenly" or "celestial").

Chanel is a female given name of French origin meaning "narrow as a pipe".

Chante is a female given name of French origin meaning "being sung".

Charisma is a female given name of Greek origin that means "blessing." Also, *charisma* is an English word meaning "compelling attractiveness or charm that can inspire devotion in others."

Cherilyn (SHER-a-lin) is a rarely used feminine given name of French origin that means "dear".

Cheryl is a female given name of French origin meaning "darling, beloved".

Chloe is a female given name. derived from the ancient Greek Khloe, means "blooming." The name is thought to be an epithet of the Greek goddess of agriculture and fertility, Demeter.

Christina is a female given name of Latin origin meaning "Christian woman".

Claire (a French form of *Clara*) is a female given name of Latin origin meaning "bright and clear".

Claudette is a female given name of Latin origin meaning "feeble woman". It is the feminine form of *Claudius*. In Roman mythology, Claudia was one of the Vestal Virgins, priestess of Vesta, Roman goddess of the hearth.

Colette is a female given name of French origin meaning "Victorious".

Constance is a feminine given name. The English word *constance* is borrowed from the French via the Latin *constantem* (meaning "steadfast, resolute, faithful"). As a female given name, the Norman-French introduced it to the English after the Conquest of 1066. In fact, one of William the Conqueror's own daughters was named Constance (later the Duchess of Brittany). The female Constance developed in medieval France probably in homage to *Constantine the Great* (272-337), the first Roman Emperor to adopt Christianity as the official state religion in the 4th century.

Cora is a given name, derived from the Greek *Koré*, the maiden name of the Greek-roman goddess Persephone (daughter of Zeus and Demeter).

Homer describes her as the formidable, venerable, majestic queen of the underworld, who carries into effect the curses of men upon the souls of the dead. She becomes the queen of the underworld through her abduction by and subsequent marriage to Hades, the god of the underworld). It was not used as a given name in the English-speaking world until after it was employed by James Fenimore Cooper for a character in his novel "The Last of the Mohicans" (1826).

Cornelia (kor-NEEL-yah) is a female given name; a feminine version of the name *Cornelius* or *Cornelis*. In the 2nd century BC, the name was borne by *Cornelia*

Scipionis Africana (the daughter of the military hero Scipio Africanus), the mother of the two reformers known as the *Gracchi*. After her death, she was regarded as an example of the ideal Roman woman. The name was revived in the 18th century.

Daenerys is a feminine given name, probably originated from *Daen* (Hebrew for "God is my judge") and *Erys* (Greek for *Eris*, goddess of discord and destruction). Daenerys would, therefore, mean "god is the judge of my destruction."

Dakota is a female name of Native American origin meaning "friendly one." Dakota derived from the name of the indigenous Native American tribe Dakota people, or from the name of two states in the United States, North Dakota and South Dakota, which are also derived from the Dakota people local to that area.

Danica (DAH-nee-tza) is an Eastern European female name. In Slavic mythology, Danica was the "daystar" and the younger sister of the Sun. She was revered among the Slavs in their ancient polytheistic religions prior to the arrival of Christianity. Danica was one of the guardian goddesses who guarded over Simargl, a dog-like creature chained to the star Polaris to prevent him from consuming the constellation and putting an end to the universe. Each morning, Danica – the Morning Star – opened the gates to the Sun's palace to release the deity across the sky and would then close the gates behind him upon return at night. The ancient Slavs prayed to her each morning at daybreak. Danica was often portrayed as a warrior goddess and a protector. In some accounts, Danica, along with her counterpart (the Evening Star), married the moon god and gave birth to all of the stars.

Darina is a female given name of Slavic origin meaning "present".

Davina (dah-VEE-nah) is a feminine given name of Scottish and Hebrew origin that means "beloved."

Delaney (da-LAY-nee) is a transferred use of a surname, originating out of England but with French (Norman) roots that means "from the alder grove" (also possibly (Irish, Gaelic) "angel from heaven"). The alder is a flowering plant from the birch family. The ancient Celtic people believed the alder had sacred giving and nurturing qualities, mainly due to its root system which provided rich nutrients back into the soil thus restoring poor ground conditions. The alder's root system can also be submerged in watery areas, so the Celts believed their roots provided shelter to fish and their decomposed leaves in the water gave rich nutrients to all water creatures. The alder wood was used by the Celtic people for crafting of musical instruments as well as an effective source of charcoal fuel. Lastly, the Celtic people believed that the alder possessed a secret, sacred flame within itself. Much revered was this plant to the ancient Celts - filled with sacred, hidden powers and a giving, restorative nature.

Desiree is a girl's name of French origin meaning "desired, wished."

Dhara is a feminine given name of Hindi origin meaning "Earth."

Edith (EE-dith) is one of the few Old English female names that survived the Norman Conquest of 1066. Originally rendered as *Eadgyð*, Edith is ultimately derived from the elements *ead* (meaning "riches, prosperity") and *gyð* (meaning "war, strife"). Edith was the illegitimate daughter of the 10th century King of England, Edgar the Peaceful. The name became rare after the 15th century but was revived in the 19th century.

Echo is a female given name of Greek origin meaning "woman of sound". In Greek mythology, Echo was a mountain nymph who was in love with her voice and could sing and play many musical instruments.

Eilish is an Irish variant of the name *Elizabeth*, which itself means "pledged to God." Also has the lesser-used variant forms of *Eilis*, *Elis*, and *Elish*.

Eira (ay-ra) is a female given name of Welsh origin meaning "snow."

Elara is a feminine given name of Greek origin. According to mythology, Elara was the daughter of King Orchomenus and mother of Tityos. She was one of Zeus' lovers and he hid her from his wife, Hera, by placing her deep beneath the earth. This was where she gave birth to Tityas, a giant who is sometimes said to be the son of Gaia, the earth goddess, for this reason. It is further added that Elara died in labor because of the enormous size of her baby. The cave through which Tityos was believed to have come to the surface of Earth was located on Euboea and referred to as *Elarion.*

Eleanor (EL-a-nor) is a feminine given name. It was the name of a number of women of the high nobility in Western Europe during the High Middle Ages, originally from a Provençal name *Aliénor* (from the Germanic *aljis,* meaning "other, foreign" (from the Proto-

Indo-European root *al,* meaning "beyond")). Eleanor is a name made popular by *Eleanor of Aquitaine* (c. 1122-1204), who was the queen of Louis VII, the king of France, and later Henry II, the king of England and one of the most glamorous, wealthy, powerful and adventurous women in all of medieval Europe. If "celebrity" were a word in the English dictionary in the 12th century, she may very well have been the poster girl definition. The popularity of the name Eleanor in England during the Middle Ages was due to the fame of Eleanor of Aquitaine, as well as two queens of the following century: *Eleanor of Provence*, the wife of Henry III, and *Eleanor of*

Castile, the wife of Edward I. More recently, it was borne by first lady *Eleanor Roosevelt* (1884-1962), the wife of American president Franklin Roosevelt. Variants of this name include *Elinor*, *Ellinor*, *Elenor*, *Eleanore*, *Eleanour*, and *Eleonora*.

Eliana (el-ee-AH-nah) is a female given name of Hebrew origin meaning "God has answered." It may also be related to the Greek *elios* (meaning "god of the sun"), and the name may thus mean "daughter of the sun." In Arabic, it is translated as "the bright."

Emberlynn (emb-erly-nn) is a female given name of English-

American origin meaning "as precious as a beautiful jewel."

Emma is a female given name of Germanic origin meaning "universal woman".

Emmeline (or *Emmaline,* or *Ameline*) (EM-a-leen) is a female given name. The medieval name, a short form of Germanic names beginning with the element *amal* (meaning "work"). It was introduced to England by the Normans.

Erina is a female given name of Latin origin meaning "the beautiful one".

Essie is a feminine name that means "myrtle", "bride", or "star." Essie is an alternate spelling of *Estelle* (Old French, Latin), and is also a variation of *Esther* (Persian).

Eternity is a rarely used feminine name derived from the English word "eternity" (meaning "existence without end; infinite time; forever").

Ethel (ETH-el) is an Old English word meaning "noble." It was coined in the 19th century, when many Old English names were revived. It was popularized by the novels "The Newcomes" (1855) by William Makepeace Thackeray and "The Daisy Chain" (1856) by C. M. Yonge. A famous bearer was

American actress and singer *Ethel Merman* (1908-1984).

Evangeline (ee-van-ja-LEEN) is a bizarre derivation of the Latin word *evangelium* (meaning "gospel"), from the Greek *euangelion* (*eu* (meaning "good") + *angelma* (meaning "tidings")). The name was brought to life by the American poet Henry Wadsworth Longfellow in his 1847 epic poem "Evangeline, A Tale of Acadie." The poem tells the story of a French girl Evangeline from the prosperous New French colonies around the maritime provinces of eastern Quebec, Canada and modern-day Nova Scotia and Maine (an area then known as Acadia). In the mid-18th century, the British fought the French and expelled these people from their land. During this Great Upheaval, Evangeline is searching for her lost love Gabriel. She wanders across the rustic scenery of America devoting her entire life to finding the man she loves. The poem was based on a true story and had a powerful effect in defining both Acadian history and identity in the nineteenth and twentieth centuries. *Evangeline* also served to identify and define the history and enduring spirit of the Acadian people. This lovely, tragic heroine was also the inspiration behind Robbie Robertson's well-known song

"Evangeline" he wrote as a duet performed by The Band and Emmylou Harris.

Everly is a female name taken from a patronymic Anglo-Saxon surname derived from a pre-11th century Old English masculine name *Eoforheard* from the Old High German *Eberhard*, meaning "brave as a wild boar", composed of the Germanic elements *eber* (wild boar) and *hard* (hardy, brave, strong).

Faith is a female given name of Latin origin meaning "trusting, believing".

Felicia is a female given name of Latin origin meaning "fortunate woman". It is a feminine form of *Felicius*, ultimately derived from Felix.

Felicity is a female given name of Latin origin meaning "filled with happiness". Felicity was the name of a 2nd century Christian saint.

Fionnuala (FINN-oola) is a feminine given name of Irish origin that means "fair shoulder" from Irish *fionn* (white, fair) and *guala* (shoulder). In Irish legend ("Children of Lir"), the chieftan King Lir and his wife Aobh had a daughter Fionnoula and three sons Aedh, Conn, and Fiachra. When Aodh died, Lir's new wife Aoife was so jealous of her husband's love for his children that she cast a spell on them and turned them into swans and condemned them to spend 300 years on Lake Daravarragh, 300 years on the Sea of Moyle and 300 years on Innis Glora. Lir pleaded with Aoife to reverse the spell, but Aoife refused. Lir became very angry and banished her from his kingdom. Until his death, Lir spent all his time beside the lake talking to his children and listening to their singing.

After three hundred years had passed they moved to the sea of Moyle between Ireland and Scotland. It was very cold and stormy on the sea. When the time came they flew to Inis Glora, by now the swans had grown old and tired. Life was easier on the island, it was warmer and there was lots of food. Then one morning they heard the sound they had been waiting for. It was the sound of a Christian church bell. They swam to shore. Outside the church where the bells were ringing was a monk named Caomhog. He was stunned when he saw the four swans turn into four old people in front of him. Fionnuala put her arms around her brothers, they were so happy to be human again. They were now 900 years old. Caomhog listened to their sad story and baptized them, soon after they died of old age. He buried them in one grave. After a while, he dreamed that he saw four children flying up through the clouds. He knew that the children of Lir were now with their father and mother.

The name is anglicized as *Fenella*. The shortened version *Nuala* is commonly used as a first name in contemporary Ireland.

Flavia (FLAH-vee-ah) is a female given name of Latin origin that means "yellow hair; blonde."

Fleur is a female given name, simply translating as "flower". Another variation is the name *Fleurine*.

Florence (FLOR-ens) is an English and French female name derived from the Latin *florens* (meaning "flourishing, blooming"). We know the masculine name *Florentius* dates back to ancient times, as it was borne by several early Christian saints in the first centuries of the Common Era. Both *Florentius* and *Florentia* were commonly used among Roman citizens especially after the Christianization of Europe (in honor of the early saints). The name can also be given in reference to the city in Italy, as in the case of *Florence Nightingale* (1820-1910). She was a nurse in British hospitals during the Crimean War and is usually considered the founder of modern nursing.

Francesca (fran-CHESS-kah) is the Italian feminine form of *Francis*. The masculine given name Francis comes from the Late Latinate *Franciscus*, a vocabulary word denoting "French" or "Frenchman." The most famous bearer was the beautiful *Francesca di Rimini* (13th century), daughter of Giovanni da Polenta, Count of Ravenna. Her love story has been retold in Dante's "Inferno."

Freya (FRAY-ə) is a female name of Norse origin meaning "lady, mistress, noblewoman." This was the name of the goddess of love, beauty, war, and death in Norse mythology. She claimed half of the heroes who were slain in battle and brought them to her realm of Fólkvangr.

Frida is a feminine given name of Old German origin; the Scandinavian form is *Fríða*. This name derived from the Germanic element *frid* (meaning "peace"). In fact, the modern word "peace" replaced the Old English *frið* which was also associated with the word "happiness" (as in peace of mind). The name was most famously borne by the celebrated Mexican painter *Frida Kahlo* (1907-1954).

Gaia is a feminine given name of Greek origin meaning "earth mother." In Greek mythology, Gaia was the mother goddess who presided over the earth.

According to one version of the Greek myth of creation, Gaia, Chaos, and Eros co-existed at the beginning of time. Another myth states that these three entities emerged out of a Cosmic Egg. The best-known myth about Gaia, however, may be found in Hesiod's *Theogony*, a poem describing the origin of the gods. In this literary work, Gaia is said to have arisen after Chaos. Gaia then gave birth to Ouranos, the personification of the Sky, whom she took as a consort. Gaia also gave birth (by herself) to Ourea (the Mountains) and Pontus (the Sea).

Genevieve (JEN-a-veev) is a French name with either Germanic or Celtic roots. An earlier version of the name, *Genovefa*, is said to come from the Germanic elements *keno* (meaning "kin") and *wefa* (meaning "wife"). Alternatively, Genevieve is probably a heavily mutated word from the Gaulish (early variety of Celtic) language elements meaning "people, tribe" and "woman." This name was borne by *Saint Genevieve*, the patron saint of Paris, who inspired the city to resist the Huns in the 5th century. When she was seven, Geneviève was induced by Bishop St. Germain of Auxerre to dedicate herself to the religious life. On the death of her parents, she moved to Paris, where she was noted for her piety and acts of charity. She had numerous prophetic visions and is said to have predicted the invasion of the Huns. When Attila threatened Paris in 451, she persuaded the inhabitants to remain and pray, assuring them that the attack would be inconsequential and that they had the protection of heaven. Attila's army went on to Orléans, 110 km (70 miles) from Paris, and was defeated. Geneviève is reported to have had great influence over King Childeric I of the Salian Franks and, in 460, to have had a church built over the tomb of St. Denis, a patron saint of France.

She was buried in the Church of the Holy Apostles, popularly known as the Church of Sainte-Geneviève. During the French Revolution in 1793, her body was burned on the Place de Grève; the relics were enshrined in the Church of Saint-Étienne-du-Mont, where they still attract pilgrims. She is often depicted with a loaf of bread to represent her generosity.

Georgia is a female given name of Old English origin meaning "worker of the earth".

Giselle (je-ZELL) is a variant of the French female name *Gisèle* which comes from the Germanic word *gisíl* (meaning "pledge"). The name is thought to be derived from the medieval practice of leaving children in foreign courts to be brought up as "pledges" for an alliance. Gisèle was the wife of Duke Rollo (Rolf) of Normandy in the 10th century. Rollo was a Viking leader to whom the lands of Normandy were granted by France's King Charles III under the provisions of a treaty after Rollo's defeat in Paris. Gisèle, the king's daughter, was also part of the compromise. Also, "Giselle" is a romantic ballet in two acts. It was first performed by the Ballet du Théâtre de l'Académie Royale de Musique at the Salle Le Peletier in Paris,

France on Monday, 28 June 1841, with Italian ballerina Carlotta Grisi as Giselle. The ballet was an unqualified triumph. Giselle became hugely popular and was staged at once across Europe, Russia, and the United States. The traditional choreography that has been passed down to the present day derives primarily from the revivals staged by Marius Petipa during the late 19th and early 20th centuries for the Imperial Ballet in St. Petersburg. Though this name became known in the English-speaking world due to ballet "Giselle" (1841), it was not regularly used until the 20th century.

Grace is a female given name of Old English origin meaning "God's favour".

Gwendoline is a female given name of Welsh origin meaning "white ring".

Gwyneth is a female given name, a form of Welsh *gwyn* (meaning "white, fair, or blessed"). It has been common in Wales since the 19th century.

Hadley (HAD-lee) is the transferred use of an Anglo-Saxon surname originating as a place name. The name is derived from the Old English words *hǣd* (meaning "heather") and *lēah* (meaning "clearing") to denote the features of the particular landscape.

Harriet (HARE-ee-et) is a female name; an English version of the French *Henriette*, a female form of *Henri*. The male name *Harry* was formed in a similar way from *Henry*. All these names are derived from *Henrik*, which is ultimately derived from the Germanic name *Heimiric*, derived from the word elements *heim* (home) and *ric* (meaning "power, ruler"). The male name Henry was first used in England by Normans. Harriet became quite common as a feminine form of Henry/Harry in the 18th century through the early 20th century. Popular nicknames for Harriet include *Hattie*, *Hatty*, *Hetty*, *Hettie*, *Hennie*, *Harry*, *Harri*, *Harrie*, and *Etta* or *Ettie*. The name can be lengthened to *Harrietta* or *Henriette*.

Hazel is a female name derived from the name of the hazelnut tree, which is derived from the Old English *hæsel* (hazel). Alternatively, the name can also be derived from the Hebrew *hazā'ēl* (God sees).

Helga (HEL-gah) is a given name, which developed as the feminine equivalent of *Helgi*, an Old Norse masculine name from *heilagr* (meaning "blessed, holy" or "the sacred one"). *Helgi Hjörvarðsson* was the son of a Norwegian king, Hjörvarðr, and his fourth wife Sigrlinn, considered the most beautiful woman in all of Scandinavia. The name was in use in England before the Norman Conquest, but appears to have died out afterwards. It was re-introduced to English-speaking nations in the 20th century from Germany and the Nordic countries. Eastern Slavic name *Olga* is derived from it.

Hermione (her-MY-oh-nee) is an ancient Greek female given name, derived from Hermes, the ancient Greek messenger god. Hermes' etymology is up for debate, but there are three common theories: either it's derived from the Greek hermeneus (meaning "the interpreter" (given Hermes' role as a messenger or interpreter between the divine and mortal worlds)). Or it may come from herma, which is a pile of stones or a manmade shrine (a cairn), usually erected along roadsides (Hermes was also the god of travelers). Even the ancient Greek philosopher Plato had a theory: that Hermes comes from eirein (meaning "the power of speech" (since he was also the god of orators)).

In Greek mythology, Hermione was the only daughter of King Menelaus of Sparta and the very beautiful Helen of Troy. Homer describes her this way in The Odyssey: "... but the gods gave no more children to Helen once she had borne her first and only child, the lovely Hermione, with the beauty of Aphrodite the golden." She was obviously quite the prize, because Hermione is often depicted in one of those ancient Greek love triangles. Apparently, her father had promised her to Pyrrhus (son of Achilles) during the Trojan War. But Orestes (son of Agamemnon and Clytemnestra) claimed her as his own bride-to-be (before the Trojan War, Hermione's grandfather had betrothed her to Orestes). A deadly battle over the girl ensued and Pyrrhus was eventually slain.

Hermione is also the name of the wife of Leontes in Shakespeare's play "The

Winter's Tale" (1610). It is now closely associated with the character Hermione Granger from the Harry Potter series of books, first released in 1997. This name is used with moderate frequency in England, although we cannot find her on the naming charts of other English-speaking nations.

Imogen is an extremely rare and unique female given name. It is the name of a princess in the play "Cymbeline" (1609) by Shakespeare. He based her on a legendary character named *Innogen*, but the name was printed incorrectly and never corrected (the name Innogen is probably derived from Gaelic *inghean* (meaning "maiden")).

In Shakespeare's play, Imogen is a beautiful, faithful and virtuous princess. In true Shakespearean style, Imogen falls in love, is forbidden from seeing her only true love, stays virtuous and true for her banished lover, is wrongfully accused of being unfaithful to him, is the target of two ill-conceived murder plots, dresses up like a man to disguise her identity, is taken in by her long-lost brothers, and is finally reunited with her man.

Iowa is a female given name of Hebrew origin meaning "beautiful land".

Irma is a female given name that comes from the Old High German *irmin* (meaning "world"). It began to be regularly used in the English-speaking world in the 19th century. It is also used in combination with other names in the abbreviated form "Irm", for example, *Irmine*, *Irmela*, *Irmgard*, *Irmgardis*, and *Irmentraud*.

Jade is a female given name, derived from an ornamental stone *Jade* used commonly in jewelry and art that is still highly valued in Asian countries. In fact, Chinese emperors were once buried in this stone in the belief it would grant them eternal life.

Jameelah (ja-MEE-lah) is a rarely used feminine name of

Arabic origin that means "beautiful."

Josephine (JOH-sa-feen) is a female given name. It is the feminine form of the name *Joseph*, which is taken from the Hebrew name *Yosef*. The original Hebrew name translates to "(God) shall add (another son)." This is a fitting translation, as Joseph was the eleventh son of Israel (Jacob) from the book of Genesis. It was originally a diminutive form of the French name *Joséphe*, and eventually became the standard form in the 19th century, replacing Joséphe, which eventually became a very rare name. The name started gaining popularity after 1800 due to the high profile of *Josephine de Beauharnais*, a French noblewoman who became Napoleon's mistress, and later his wife. *Josette* is one of the rare and beautiful variations of Josephine.

Judith is a female given name of Hebrew origin meaning "Judea woman". It is a feminine form of *Judah*. Judith was a character in the Book of Genesis. She is also the heroine of the Book of Judith, a part of the Old Testament.

Juliana is a female given name of Latin origin meaning "soft-haired".

Kaiya is a feminine given name of Japanese origin that means "forgiveness."

Katherine (or *Catherine*) (KATH-rin, KATH-er-rin) is a feminine given name. The name originated from the Greek *Aikaterina* or *Aikaterinē*, which is of uncertain etymology. The earliest known use of the Greek name is in reference to *Saint Catherine* of *Alexandria*. The theory that the name comes from *Hecate*, the name of the Greek goddess of magic, is regarded by the editors of the Oxford Dictionary of First Names as unconvincing. In the early Christian era, it came to be associated with the Greek adjective *katharos* (meaning "pure"), leading to the alternative spellings *Katharine* and *Katherine*. The former spelling, with a middle _a_, was more common in the past and is currently more popular in the United States than in Britain. Katherine, with a middle _e_, was first recorded in England in 1196 after being brought back from the Crusades.

Kiara (kee-AR-ah) is a feminine given name that can be a variation of the Italian name *Chiara* (meaning "bright"), or the Irish name *Ciara* (meaning "dark-haired"), or the Hindi name *Kiara* (meaning "god's precious gift").

Kimberly is a female given name of Old English origin meaning "Cyneburg's clearing". It refers to Kimberley, a city is South Africa, named after Lord Kimberley.

Kira (a variant of *Ciara*) is a female given name of Irish origin meaning "little dark girl".

Kristina (kriss-TEEN-ah) is the German, Scandinavian, Slavic, and Russian form of *Christina*, which itself is a feminized version of the Medieval Latin name *Christianus* (meaning quite obviously "a Christian"). Names like *Christian*, *Christiana*, *Christina*, and *Christine* have been in use since the middle Ages but did not become widely common until the 17th century.

Lane is a female given name of English origin meaning "from a narrow lane". It was derived from an old English surname and as a surname it functions until today.

Lara is a female given name, a diminutive of *Larissa*. Larissa originates in Greek language and means "woman from citadel".

Lauren is a female given name of Latin origin meaning "laurel tree". It is a feminine form of Laurence. It is taken from the name of an aromatic evergreen large shrub. In the Greco-

Roman era, laurel was used as a symbol of victory, fame and honor.

Layana is a Persian name for girls that means "radiant", "shining", "glowing", figuratively meaning "beautiful".

Lea is a female given name, originated from Biblical times, wherein Hebrew, the name Leah meant "wearied". This may have been due to Jacob's wife in the Old Testament, Leah, giving birth to seven sons to her husband who only married her under duress. That said, the name translates to various meanings across several cultures. In Irish, Leah means "the light of the sun," or the name means "glad tidings" in Greek or "mistress, or ruler" in Assyrian.

Leila (LAY-lah) is a feminine given name in the Hebrew and Arabic languages. In Arabic, *Leila* means "night."
Arabs would use this name for their daughters in the convention of describing the quality or character of the baby; as such it has come to mean "dark beauty" or "one who was born at night." The name has been in use since medieval times inspired by the true Arabian legend of "Qays and Layla" - a story of unrequited love. These young virgin lovers fall so deeply in love that they are barely able to contain their devotion.

Causing quite the scandal in their community, Qays is denied her hand in marriage and kept from seeing her. He flees the tribe, wanders in the wilderness chanting love poems about his darling Layla, eventually descends into madness and finally dies. It is more commonly thought of as an internationally adopted name at this point as evidenced by the growing number of spelling variations: *Layla*, *Laila*, *Laylah* and *Lailah* for instance. The variant of Leila is perhaps the oldest in the English-speaking world, introduced by Lord Byron in the early 19th century as a character in his poems "The Giaour" (1813) and "Don Juan" (1819).

Leona is the female equivalent to *Leon*. Leon comes from the Greek *leon* (meaning "lion"). Leona is most popular in the nation of Croatia today. The French form of Leona is *Leonie*.

Letty is a female given name, a diminutive of *Letitia*. Letitia originates in Latin language and means "happy and joyous woman".

Lilith is a feminine given name derived from word *lilitu* that means "belonging to the night." Lilith is a figure in Jewish mythology, developed earliest in the Babylonian Talmud (3rd to 5th centuries). Lilith is often envisioned as a dangerous demon of the night, who is sexually wanton, and who steals babies in the darkness. The character is generally thought to derive in part from a historically far earlier class of female demons (*lilītu*) in ancient Mesopotamian religion, found in cuneiform texts of Sumer, the Akkadian Empire, Assyria, and Babylonia. In Jewish folklore, from the satirical book Alphabet of Sirach onwards, Lilith appears as Adam's first wife, who was created at the same time (Rosh Hashanah) and from the same dirt as Adam – compare Genesis 1:27 (that contrasts with Eve, who was created from one of Adam's ribs: Genesis 2:22). The legend developed extensively during the Middle Ages, in the tradition of

Aggadah, the Zohar, and Jewish mysticism. For example, in the 13th-century writings of Isaac ben Jacob ha-Cohen, Lilith left Adam after she refused to become subservient to him and then would not return to the Garden of Eden after she had coupled with the archangel Samael. Due to the mythologies of Lilith, she has been a dark subject of many Western artistic genres ranging from paintings to gothic literature, sci-fi, horror, and the occult. Although considered pretty rare, Lilith has been used occasionally among English speakers (although often as an elaboration of the ever-popular name *Lily*).

Lina is a female given name. In Greek, Lina translates to "sunlight," while in Persian it simply means "light," and in Arabic, it means "tender."

Linnet is a female given name of French origin meaning "flaxen-haired."

Liserli is a feminine given name of Swiss origin meaning "God's Oath." Also, there is a similar name **Lisali**, of African origin, meaning "light."

Lorelei (LOR-a-lye) is a feminine given name with two etymologies. First, it's the combination of an Old German word *lureln* (meaning "murmuring") + a Celtic word *ley* (meaning "rock"). Second, it could be derived from the Germanic *lauern* (meaning "to lurk or lie in wait") along with the aforementioned Celtic word for rock. Therefore, the name either means "murmuring rock" or "lurking rock." Lorelei is the name of a rock positioned on the banks of the Rhine, a European river flowing from Switzerland to the North Sea. The Lorelei (or *Loreley*) rock is located at the narrowest point of the river and is therefore subjected to strong currents and rocky conditions which have caused scores of maritime accidents (the heavy currents create the "murmuring" sound owing to the rock's name). As such, various legends concerning the dangerous rock have sprung up around Lorelei by German poets (the rock is located on a portion of the river located in Germany). For example, one of such legends says that a maiden named the Lorelei lives on the rock and lures fishermen to their death with her song.

Louise is thought to be of Old German origin, translating to "famous warrior." Louise is the feminized version of *Louis* and the French name *Ludwig*.

Luciana is a feminine given name of Roman origin, a variation of the masculine name *Lucius*, from the Latin *lux* (meaning "light"). Like Marcus and Julius, Lucius is one of the oldest and most common Roman given names dating back to the now-extinct Etruscan civilization. Due to the name's etymological meaning (i.e., "light"), Lucius was often bestowed upon children who were born at the first light of dawn (which would explain the heavy usage).

Luna (LOO-nah) is a female given name derived from the Latin *luna* (the moon). She was the Roman mythological goddess of the moon and is equated with the Greek *Selene* (goddess of the moon; daughter of the Titans Hyperion and Theia, and sister of the sun-god Helios, and goddess of the dawn, Eos). Closely mapping her

Greek incarnation, Luna rode her white chariot across the sky wearing the moon as her crown to illuminate the night as she traveled to be with her mortal husband Endymion. She was an important deity to the Romans since they depended upon the moon for calculating the time (i.e., the lunar calendar).

Lyra (LEE-ra) is a female given name derives from the Greek *lýra* (meaning "a lyre").

Madeleine is a feminine given name. It is a form of *Magdalene*, well-known because of *Saint Mary Magdalene*. In the United States, this name often appears under the spelling *Madeline*. Magdalene means "from

Magdala." Mary Magdalene's name is thought to be derived from *Magdala* (a village on the sea of Galilee). In Aramaic, *magdala* means "tower" or "elevated, great, magnificent." Additionally, in German, *Mädelein* means "little girl."

Maeve is a feminine given name of Irish origin meaning "she who intoxicates".

Magdalena is a female given name of Biblical origin meaning "Gift of God".

Maisie is a female given name of Old English origin meaning "Child of light" or "pearl".

Manon is a French version of *Madeline* and is considered to mean "wished-for child", though it has also been posited that Manon is a diminutive of Marie. The name has proven most popular in France and Belgium, though the names Marie and Madeline (to which it is closely related) are more broadly popular across the United Kingdom and other European countries.

Marcella is a feminine given name of Latin origin, a variation of the masculine name *Marcellus* (meaning "belonging to Mars").

Margaux is a female given name meaning "pearl" (derived

from the Greek *maragon*), the name Margaux is both a version of *Margaret* and *Margot*. It can also translate to Margarid and Margarit (Armenian), Margarita (Bulgarian), Margareta (Croation), Margreet (Dutch) and Marjorie in English.

Marguerite (Mar-gu-reet) is a rare female name that can be a variation of the name *Margaret* (a female first name, derived from the noun *margaron* (meaning "pearl")). Marguerite is also the French word for the daisy flower (species Leucanthemum vulgare).

Marianna (mahr-YAHN-nah) is a feminine given name. Firstly, way back in the Middle

Ages, the female name Marian developed as a variant of *Marion* which was a French diminutive of *Marie*. The Norman-French brought Marion to England after the Norman Conquest in the 11th century where it was adopted as *Marian* (as evidenced by *Maid Marian* in the Tales of Robin Hood). Marianna could have been created later as an embellished form of Marian. Secondly, Marianna came into vogue in the late 19th century due to a fashionable trend which was emerging at the time whereby separate female names were combined to create one new name (Marianna = Mary + Anna). Lastly, Marianna is the English form of the Spanish

Mariana which may have developed as the female form of an Old Roman family name *Marianus* – itself coming from either *Mars* (the Roman god of war) or the Latin word *mas* (meaning "sea").

Marishka is a rare female name that can be a variation of the name *Mary*, the mother of Jesus, a symbol of pure and deep love, but the meaning of the name is disputed; maybe it means "bitterness." Another possibility is an Egyptian origin with the name derived from *mry* (beloved).

Medina is a female name derived from several cities and towns of Spain such as *Medina* *del Campo*, *Medina de Pomar*, *Medina de Rioseco*, *Medinaceli*, *Medina-Sidonia*, *Medina de las Torres* and many others. The use of the term dates back to the Muslim rule of Al Andalus (8th–15th century) and it originates from the Arabic word *madīnah* (means "city").

Meira is a feminine given name of Hebrew origin meaning "light." It is a feminine form of *Meir*.

Melania is a feminine given name (a version of *Melanie*) of Greek origin that means "black, dark."

Melina (ma-LEEN-ah) is a female name of Greek origin

that comes from the Greek word for "honey." *Mel* can be derived from names such as *Melanie* (meaning "god's gift") or *Melissa* (meaning "honey-bee").

Mercedes is a female given name of Spanish origin meaning "gracious gifts, benefits".

Merindah (meh-RIN-da) is a feminine given name that means "beautiful" in one of the Indigenous languages of the Sydney area.

Mikaela (mi-khah-E-lah, mi-KAY-la) is the Scandinavian and Finnish spelling of *Michaela*, which itself is the female equivalent of the masculine name *Michael*. The name

Michael originated from the Hebrew word *mikha'el*, which actually translates into a question: "Who is like God?" Mikaela is also a form of *Michelle* (French, Hebrew).

Mila is a female given name, an abbreviated version of names beginning or ending in *Mila* (Milada, Milena or Ludmila). The name Ludmila is formed by the elements *lud* (meaning people) and *mila* (meaning dear, love).

Mileva is a feminine given name of Slavic, Czech, Bulgarian origin meaning "gracious, dear."

Mirabelle is a female given name that comes from the Latin word *mirabilis* (meaning "wonderful"). This name was coined during the Middle Ages, though it eventually died out. It was briefly revived in the 19th century, but again the name was quietly forgotten.

Morwenna (moor-WEE-nuh) is a very beautiful, magical name. There are many meanings given for it, but most seem to come from people trying to find Welsh/Cornish words it looks like. It's most likely that *mor* means "sea" and the rest is just unknown. It certainly doesn't mean "maiden" in Cornish, as that is "moren."

Muriel is an English female given name derived from Celtic elements *muir* (meaning "sea") and *gheal* (meaning "bright").

Myra (MYE-rah) is a feminine given name created by the 17th-century poet Fulke Greville. He possibly based it on Latin *myrra* (meaning "myrrh" (a fragrant resin obtained from a tree)). Otherwise, he may have simply rearranged the letters from the name *Mary*. Although unrelated etymologically, this is also the name of an ancient city of Anatolia. Also, Myra may have been influenced by the name *Miranda*, from the Latin *mirari* (meaning "to wonder at, to admire"). Aside from Myra's literary connection to the poetry of Greville, Myra is sometimes considered a female form of

Myron, which also comes from the Greek word for *myrrh* (meaning "sweet perfume").

Naomi is a female given name of Old English origin meaning "pleasant" or "beautiful".

Nereida is a female given name derived from Greek *Nereides* (meaning "nymphs, sea sprites"), ultimately derived from the name of the Greek sea god Nereus, who supposedly fathered them. Nereus, in Greek religion, sea god called by Homer "Old Man of the Sea," noted for his wisdom, gift of prophecy, and ability to change his shape. He was the son of Pontus, a personification of the sea, and Gaea, the Earth goddess. The Nereids (water nymphs) were his daughters by the Oceanid Doris, and he lived with them in the depths of the sea, particularly the Aegean. Aphrodite, the goddess of love, was his pupil.

Nicolina is a feminine form of *Nicolas*, which is from the Greek *Nikolaos*, a compound name composed of the elements *nikē* (victory) and *laos* (the people): hence, "victory of the people".

Nina is a female given name of Russian origin meaning "mighty" or "fire".

Nixie is a female given name, probably derived from a Germanic name for water spirits and sprites who appear in human form.

Nora is a female given name of Latin origin meaning meaning "honor".

Octavia (ock-TAHV-yah, ock-TAY-vee-ah) is a female given name of Latin origin that means "eighth." Octavia was the wife of Mark Antony and the sister of Roman emperor Augustus. In 19th-century England, this name was sometimes given to the eighth-born child.

Olympia is a female given name, a form of Olympos, which originates in Greek language and is derived from Mount

Olympus, the highest mountain in Greece.

Ophelia is a female given name of Greek origin meaning "helpful woman". It was popularized by William Shakespeare in his tragedy Hamlet.

Pandora is a feminine given name of Greek origin meaning "all gifted"; name derivated from Pandora, the first woman according to Greek mythology. According to Hesiod's Theogony, after Prometheus, a fire god and divine trickster, had stolen fire from heaven and bestowed it upon mortals, Zeus, the king of the gods, determined to counteract this blessing. He accordingly commissioned

Hephaestus (a god of fire and patron of craftsmen) to fashion a woman out of the earth, upon whom the gods bestowed their choicest gifts. In Hesiod's Works and Days, Pandora had a jar containing all manner of misery and evil. Zeus sent her to Epimetheus, who forgot the warning of his brother Prometheus and made Pandora his wife. She afterward opened the jar, from which the evils flew out over the earth. Hope alone remained inside, the lid having been shut down before she could escape. In a later story, the jar contained not evils but blessings, which would have been preserved for the human race had they not been lost through the opening of the jar out of curiosity. Pandora's jar became a box in the 16th century when the Renaissance humanist Desiderius Erasmus either mistranslated the Greek or confused the vessel with the box in the story of "Cupid and Psyche".

Parisa is a female given name of Persian origin meaning "fairy-like". It is a popular feminine given name mainly in Iran.

Paulina (pawl-EEN-ah) is a feminine given name. It is a female version of *Paulinus*, a variant of *Paulus* (meaning "the little"). The name came into use among English-speaking countries in the 19th century. Other versions of this name include *Paula* (English, Spanish), *Paola* (Italian), *Pauline* (French, German and Scandinavian), *Paulette* (French), and *Polina* (Russian).

Payton (or *Peyton*) is a female given name of Old English origin meaning "from the town of Paega".

Penelope is a female given name, adopted from Greek mythology for the wife of Odysseus, *Penelopē*, who spent time weaving while she waited 20 years for her husband's return from the Trojan War. The etymology of the name is debated. Some believe it is derived from the Greek *penelops* (a kind of duck), since Penelope was said to have been exposed to die as an infant and was fed and protected by a duck. Others think it might be derived from *pēnē* (thread on a bobbin) and give it the definition "weaver, a worker of the loom," for Penelope spent evenings weaving and unweaving while she waited for her husband to return. The name has since been associated with "faithfulness."

Photine is a female given name of Ancient Greek origin, meaning "enlightened one, light, brilliant." The holy and glorious *Great-martyr Photine of Samaria* (also *Photini* or *Svetlana*), Equal-to-the-Apostles, encountered Christ at the well of Jacob. Tradition relates that the Apostles baptized her with the name "Photine", meaning "enlightened one."

Priscilla (pri-SIL-ə or pree-SHEEL-la (Italian)) is a female given name, a diminutive form of the Latin *Prisca*, a feminine form of *Priscus*, which is a Roman surname derived from *priscus* (meaning "ancient"). The name appears in English literature in Edmund Spenser's "The Faerie Queene" (1596) and was adopted as an English name by the Puritans in the 17th century. Henry Wadsworth Longfellow used it in his poem "The Courtship of Miles Standish" (1858).

Promise is a female given name of Old French *promesse* (meaning "Guarantee" and "Assurance").

Queenie is a female given name that comes from the English word "queen."

Rebecca (ree-BEK-ah) is a feminine given name originating from the Hebrew language. The etymology of the name is debated. The Hebrew name *Rivka* possibly means "to snare, bind, trap" but is also said to mean "captivating." Some etymologists believe the name is of Aramaic origin (an ancestral language of Arabic) meaning "soil, earth."

Regina (re-JEEN-ah) is a feminine given name that comes from the Latin language and means "queen." The name has been in use since medieval times influenced in part by *St. Regina*, a 3rd-century French saint and virgin martyr. Regina's mother died in childbirth and her pagan father rejected her. A Christian nurse took her in and baptized her. As a young woman, she was beheaded for refusing to give up her Christian faith as a stipulation of her marriage to a Roman pagan proconsul. Virgin martyrs became quite venerated in the Middle Ages and names of admired saints were given to children as a protective measure. Regina was one such example of this medieval naming trend. Aside from that, "Regina Coeli" (Queen of Heaven) became a popular Latin epithet for the Virgin Mother in the early Middle Ages. This also served to influence the name Regina centuries ago. In England, the name experienced a revival in the 19th century and spread among other English-speaking nations. Variants of this name include *Régine*, *Geena*, *Gina*, and *Jeanna*.

Reina (RAY-nah) is the Spanish word for "queen." Usage of Reina as a female given name is similar to the usage of *Regina* (Latin word for "queen") or the Celtic-Welsh *Rhiannon* (Rihanna) meaning "great queen." The words *queen* and *reina* developed from two different language families. The Spanish *reina* is derived from the Latin *regina* (which developed as a feminine form of *rex* (Latin for king)). These are both rooted in the Latin *regere* ("to rule"). On the other hand, the word "queen" comes from the Germanic branch derived from the Old English *cwēn*, which was the common word for "woman." Today we would all agree that the words Reina and Queen now mean the same thing: that is, a woman in power and one who rules.

Renata is a Late Latin female name from *Renatus* (meaning "reborn"). Renata is used mainly by the Spanish and Italians, but it is also circulated among Germans and Slavs (the French equivalent is *Renée*). Renata is essentially a Christian name bestowed upon baby girls in celebration of Jesus' resurrection; or in reference to the spiritual "rebirth" through a daughter's baptism.

Rhiannon is a feminine given name of Welsh origin meaning "divine queen." It is speculated that this was the name of an otherwise unattested Celtic goddess of fertility and the moon.

Rhosyn is a feminine given name meaning "rose" in Welsh.

Rieka is a feminine given name of Old German origin meaning "complete ruler; peaceful ruler."

Rionach (Ree-oh-nah) is a feminine given name of Irish origin meaning "queenly." In legend, Rionach was the wife of "Niall of the Nine Hostages" and as such is the maternal ancestor of many of the great Irish family dynasties.

Rosaline is a female name that has its roots in French, Old German and Latin, and means "gentle." Rosaline is a version of *Rosalie* (French) and can also mean "rose garden." This is the name of characters in Shakespeare's "Love's Labour's

Lost" (1594) and "Romeo and Juliet" (1596).

Rose is a female given name. The name of the flower derives from the Old English and the Latin "rosa". In France, both Rose and Rosalie are popular names, while the name is related to Rosalia and Rosa in Spanish, Roisin in Gaelic, Roze in Latvian, Roos in Dutch, Rosaria and Rosalia in Portuguese, and Rozalia in Slovak.

Rosemary (ROHZ-mare-ee) is a feminine given name, a combination of the names *Rose* and *Mary*. Rosemary also shares her name with the herb, from the Latin *ros* (meaning "dew") and *marinus* (meaning "sea"), resulting from the fact that rosemary, native to the Mediterranean region, needed very little water to survive. Rather, rosemary only needed the "dew of the sea" or the humidity carried from the Mediterranean breezes. As a female given name, Rosemary came into style in the 19th century when naming daughters after trees, plants and flowers became quite fashionable.

Roux is a female given name of French origin meaning "reddish brown".

Ruta is a female given name, a Polish variant of *Ruth*.

Ruth is an ancient Biblical name, from the Hebrew *re'ut* (meaning "friend, companion"). Ruth was the young Moabite widow of Mahlon who said to his Hebrew mother Naomi: "Where you go, there I shall go also; your people will be my people, your God, my God." Her sentiments appealed to Victorian poets, and the name has been popular since the 17th century.

Sabine is the French, German and Danish version of the more common name, *Sabina*. It possibly originates from the Latin word *Sabinus*, referring to the Sabines who lived in northeastern Rome.

Sabrina (sa-BREE-nah) is a feminine given name found primarily in Western European cultures and to a lesser extent in the Arabic world. According to a legend recounted by Geoffrey of Monmouth in the 12th century, *Habren* or Sabrina, the Latinized form of the river's Common Brittonic or proto-Welsh name, was the daughter of a king named Locrinus (also known as Locrin or Locrine in English) by his mistress, the Germanic princess Estrildis. Locrinus ruled England after the death of his father, Brutus of Troy, the legendary second founder of Britain. Locrinus cast aside his wife, Guendolen, and their son Maddan and acknowledged Sabrina and her mother, but the enraged Guendolen raised an army against him and defeated Locrinus in battle. Guendolen then ordered that Sabrina and her mother be drowned in the river. The river was named after Sabrina so Locrine's betrayal of Guendolen would never be forgotten. According to legend, Sabrina lives in the river, which reflects her mood. She rides in a chariot and dolphins and salmon swim alongside her. The later story suggests that the legend of Sabrina could have become intermingled with old stories of a river goddess or nymph. It was popularized as a given name by Samuel A. Taylor's play "Sabrina Fair"

(1953) and the movie adaptation that followed it the next year.

Saige is a female name of Latin origin that means "wise."

Samsara - a very unique female given name. *Saṃsāra* is a Sanskrit word for the repetitive cycle of death and rebirth. It encompasses the concept of reincarnation and the fact that what an individual does in their current life will be reflected, through karma, in their future lives. The literal translation of samsara would be "a wandering through." This refers to the way in which everyone passes through a number of lives and states.

Saoirse (SEER-sha) is a feminine name of Irish origin meaning "liberty." Given its meaning, it may well have been in response to Irish independence, which had dominated the previous decade and the early 20s. Irish-American actress *Saoirse Ronan* has helped the world to recognise (and pronounce) the name.

Selene (si-LEE-nee or SEH-LEH-NEH (in Classical Greek) is a female given name of Greek origin; it is likely connected to the word *selas*, meaning "brightness." Daughter of Greek titans Hyperion and Theia, Selene was a lunar deity who presided over the moon and all it represented: the night, the tides and fertility.

Serena (ser-REE-nah) is a female given name born from the English adjective *serene*, from the Latin *serenus* (meaning "peaceful, tranquil, calm, clear" (used initially to describe the weather and later became an adjective applied to persons)). As a female name, Serena dates back to at least the late 16th century. English poet Edmund Spenser used it in his literary masterpiece and the allegorical poem "The Faerie Queene" (Book VI). Serena is a minor character, a knight's lady, who learns the only way to overcome the Beast's poisonous venom is through virtue, honesty, and self-control (sounds like her name was not accidentally chosen by the author).

In Philippine mythology, *Sirena* is a mythological aquatic creature with the head and torso of a human female and the tail of a fish. Sirena has a beautiful and enchanting voice that can attract and hypnotize males, especially fishermen. She sings to sailors and enchants them, distracting them from their work and causing them to walk off ship decks or cause shipwrecks.

Sirens sing with enchanting voices while hiding among the rocks by the shore. When the men hear these songs they are hypnotized and are abducted by the Sirens. Some folk traditions claim that Sirens carry their victims under the sea, sacrificing them to the water deities. Other stories claim that they pretend to need rescuing from drowning, luring men into the sea, but proceed to squeeze the life out of any man who falls prey to their hoax.

Sia is a feminine Swedish given name derived from the Old Norse *sigr* (meaning "victory").

Sienna (SEE-en-uh) is a female given name that is derived from the Italian city of Siena, which gave its name to a reddish shade of brown. The name itself is possibly influenced by the word sienna, meaning "orange-red."

Sierra (see-ERR-ah) is the Spanish term for a mountain range, coming from the Latin word *serra* (meaning "saw, jagged", signifying their saw-toothed appearance). Sierra developed as a female given name in the United States, most notably in reference to the *Sierra Nevada* mountain range that straddles the California-Nevada borders and extends from California's Central Valley 400 miles north to the Mount Shasta area. This magnificent mountain range features some of the most beautiful areas known on earth, including Yosemite Valley, Mt. Whitney and Lake Tahoe. The literal translation is "snowy mountains" (from the Spanish *sierra* (a range of hills) and *nevado* (meaning "snowy").

Sigourney is a rare female name of uncertain origin. This name made famous by actress *Sigourney Weaver*, who was originally named Susan.

Simone is a female given name of Hebrew origin meaning "one who has heard".

Skylar is a female given name of Dutch origin meaning "noble scholar". Newer, simpler forms of the Dutch surname *Schuyler*; has quite a few other spelling variations out there including *Skyler* and *Skyllar*.

Sloane is a feminine given name of Irish origin meaning "raider." Sloane could also be considered a place name in reference to Sloane Square located in the chic Chelsea neighborhood of West London. The term "Sloane Ranger" was coined in the 1980s to signify the young, professional, upper-class women who lived near the Square and styled themselves after the fashionable Diana, Princess of Wales. As a female given name, Sloane has primarily been used in the United States but occasionally shows up in Canada and Australia, as well.

Sophia (or *Sonya*, as a variation) is a female given name of Greek origin meaning "woman of wisdom".

Stella is a female given name of Latin origin meaning "star".

Tereza is a female given, a Czech variant of *Theresa*, and means "summer harvest".

Thalia is a female given name, derived from the Greek *thallein* (to flourish, to bloom). In Greek mythology she was one of the nine Muses, presiding over comedy and pastoral poetry.

Tiffany is a female given name of Greek origin meaning "seeing God, vision of God".

Trinity is a female given name. The English word Trinity is derived from Latin *Trinitas* (meaning "three, a triad"). The word is most closely associated with the Christian doctrine of the Trinity which signifies the unity of the three "persons": the Father, the Son and the Holy Spirit. Essentially, together, they form the one essence of God. It has only been in use as a given name since the 20th century.

Uma is a female given name of Sanskrit origin meaning "mother".

Undine is a female given name derived from Latin word *unda* (meaning "wave"). Undines are a category of elemental beings associated with water, first named in the alchemical writings of Paracelsus. Similar creatures are found in classical literature, particularly "Ovid's Metamorphoses." Later writers developed the undine into a water nymph in its own right, and it continues to live in modern literature and art through such adaptations as Hans Christian Andersen's "The Little Mermaid." Undines are almost invariably depicted as being female and are usually found in forest pools and waterfalls. The group contains many species, including *nereides*, *limnads*, *naiades*, and *mermaids*. Although resembling humans in a form they lack a human soul, so to achieve immortality they must acquire one by marrying a human. Such a union is not without risk for the man because if he is unfaithful he is fated to die.

Ursula (UR-soo-lah) is a diminutive of *Ursa*, which is Latin for "she-bear" (as in the celestial constellations *Ursa Major* and *Ursa Minor*, aka the Big Dipper and the Little Dipper). According to Greek Mythology, Callisto was transformed into a bear by Hera when it was discovered Hera's husband, Zeus, had an affair with the beautiful nymph. That union produced a son who almost shot his bear-mother with a bow before Zeus turned him into a bear and set them both, mother and son, together in the night's sky (hence Great Bear and Little Bear).

Valerie is a female given name of Latin origin meaning "powerful, strong".

Verity (*Veretie*, *Verety*, *Verita*, *Veritie*, etc.) is a female first name and a surname. As a first name, it derives from the Latin feminine noun *veritas*, meaning "truth." It is thus an equivalent of Alethea, a female first name first used in England circa 1585, derived from the ancient and Modern Greek feminine noun *αλήθεια* (pronounced "al-ee-thia"), meaning "truth." It was adopted in England as a Puritan virtue name, truthfulness being considered as a desirable attribute especially in a female.

Victoria is a female given name of Latin origin meaning "Victory" and "Conquer".

Virginia is a feminine given name derived from the Ancient Roman family name *Virginius*; a name probably derived from the Latin word *virgo* (meaning "maiden" or "virgin"). According to myths, Virginia was a Roman girl who was killed by her father to save her from seduction by the corrupt government official Appius Claudius Crassus.

Vivian (VIV-ee-en) is a female given name of Latin origin that comes from *vivus* (meaning "alive"). Although the Normans brought the name to England after the Conquest of 1066, Vivian was popularized in England in the 19th century as a female name thanks to Lord Alfred Tennyson's "Merlin and Vivien" published in 1859. In the poem, Vivien is the duplicitous enchantress of the wizard Merlin from the Arthurian Legends. From this Celtic perspective, the name *Béibhinn* (pronounced *Vevin*) means "sweet, melodious lady" or "fair lady".

Whitney is a female given name of Old English origin meaning "from a white island". Initially, it was a surname derived from a place name.

Winona (wyw-NOH-nah) is a Native American Indian name from *Winúŋna* (meaning "firstborn daughter" or "eldest daughter" in the Sioux Dakota language). It was the name shared by both the wife and daughter of a well-known Sioux Chief, *Wapasha III* (c. 1816-1876), whose people lived on lands along the western banks of the Mississippi River in southeast Minnesota. Wabasha III, like his fathers before him, spent his life defending the land for his people in the midst of constant conflict and uprisings. Eventually they were forcibly stripped of their land and displaced to reservations in Nebraska and South Dakota. The region belonging to the

Sioux Dakotas where Wapasha III once ruled as Chief is now located in Winona County, Minnesota (named after the Chief's firstborn daughter).

Xaviera (zay-vee-EHR-ah) is a feminine form of *Xavier*, both derived from the 16th-century Roman Catholic *Saint Francis Xavier*.

Yasmin is a female given name of Persian origin meaning "jasmine flower".

Yolanda is a female given name that comes from the medieval French name *Yolande*, which was probably a form of the name *Violante*, which was itself a derivative of Latin *viola* (meaning "violet"). This name was borne by a 12th-century empress of the Latin Empire in Constantinople, who was originally from Flanders. It was also used by her descendants in the royal families of Hungary (spelled *Jolánta*) and Spain (sometimes spelled *Violante*). *The Blessed Yolanda of Poland* was a daughter of Bela IV of Hungary who married a Polish duke.

Another notable bearer was a 13th-century countess of *Vianden* in Luxembourg who joined a convent against her parents' wishes, later becoming the subject of medieval legend.

Yvette (or *Ivette*) is a female given name of Germanic origin meaning "of the yew tree".

Zelda is a female given name, a diminutive of *Griselda*. Griselda is a name of German origin that means "fighting in darkness".

Zena is a female name of Greek origin that means "guest, stranger." This name has occasionally been used since the 19th century.

Zendaya (zehn-DAY-ə) is a female name of African origin meaning "to give thanks."

Zerenity is a feminine given name of English origin meaning "calm".

Zoey is a female given name of Greek origin meaning "life".

Made in the USA
San Bernardino, CA
10 February 2020

64237305R00153